John Hunter

Observations on the Diseases of the Army in Jamaica

John Hunter

Observations on the Diseases of the Army in Jamaica

ISBN/EAN: 9783337330149

Printed in Europe, USA, Canada, Australia, Japan

Cover: Foto ©ninafisch / pixelio.de

More available books at **www.hansebooks.com**

OBSERVATIONS

ON THE

DISEASES OF THE ARMY

IN

JAMAICA.

OBSERVATIONS,

ON THE

DISEASES OF THE ARMY

IN JAMAICA;

AND ON THE

BEST MEANS OF PRESERVING THE
HEALTH OF EUROPEANS,

IN THAT CLIMATE.

BY

JOHN HUNTER, M.D. F.R.S.

AND PHYSICIAN TO THE ARMY

LONDON:
PRINTED FOR G. NICOL, PALL-MALL,
BOOKSELLER TO HIS MAJESTY.

M.DCC.LXXXVIII.

TO

SIR GEORGE BAKER, BART.
PHYSICIAN TO THEIR MAJESTIES,
PRESIDENT OF THE COLLEGE OF PHYSICIANS,
AND F. R. S.

AND

WILLIAM HEBERDEN, M.D. F.R.S.
AND FELLOW OF THE COLLEGE OF PHYSICIANS.

GENTLEMEN,

THE interest you were pleased to take in my appointment to the office, in which I had an opportunity of making the observations contained in the following pages, will be deemed, I hope, a good reason for addressing you on the present occasion. It is indeed with the greatest pleasure,

pleasure, that I seize this opportunity of acknowledging the great obligations, which I owe to your friendship. The zeal with which you have successfully laboured in the improvement of medical knowledge, is equally honourable to yourselves, and beneficial to the public. That you may long continue to set an example so worthy of imitation, must be the sincere wish of all who know you, and of none more than,

   GENTLEMEN,

    Your much obliged

    and most humble Servant,

Charles Street,
April 3d, 1786.

   JOHN HUNTER.

PREFACE.

THE following obfervations were made, while I had the care and fuperintendance of the military hofpitals in the ifland of Jamaica, from the beginning of the year 1781 till the month of May 1783.

The dreadful mortality, that has always accompanied military operations in the Weft Indies, in confequence of ficknefs and difeafe, renders every attempt to point out the caufes of fuch calamities, and the means of obviating them, an object worthy of the public attention. In treating of this ſubject, I have confined myſelf to an account of thoſe things only, that fell under my own obſervation. This I have not done, as undervaluing the labours of others; but from a conviction that in Phyſic, as in all other branches of natural knowledge, he who ſhall content himſelf with narrating what he has ſeen, will perform a work more likely to be uſeful towards the improvement of knowledge, than if he endeavoured to add to the value of his own labours, by collecting the opinions of others, which there is ſome danger of his miſtaking, or miſrepreſenting.

There is much ſimilarity among the diſeaſes of warm climates; and the *Remittent Fever* appears to be the diſorder which prevails chiefly in all of them. That

PREFACE.

That difeafe, as defcribed on the coaft of Africa *, and on the banks of the Ganges †, would feem to be nearly the fame as in Jamaica. It is therefore probable that the method of cure, which was found fuccefsful in that ifland, would anfwer equally well in thofe, or fimilar climates: but this can only be determined by experience.

* See Robertfon's Phyfical Journal kept on board his Majefty's fhip RAINBOW, Part i. chap. 1 and 2.

† See Clark's Obfervations on voyages to the Eaft Indies, p. 168, cafe vi. & feq.

CONTENTS.

CONTENTS.

Page

INTRODUCTION. Of the Situation, Face of the Country, Climate, and Produce of the Island of Jamaica - - - - 1

CHAP. I.

SECT. I. *Of the Causes of Sickness and Mortality, among Soldiers and Europeans, in Jamaica* - - - 12

SECT. II. *Of the Precautions to be taken in sending Troops to the West Indies; and of the Means of pre-*

† *serving*

CONTENTS.

Page

serving their Health in that Climate - - - - 27

CHAP. II.

Of the Number of Men lost annually by the several Regiments in Jamaica; and of the various Degrees of Healthiness of the different Quarters - - - - 39

CHAP. III.

Of Fevers - - - - 76

SECT. I. Of the Symptoms of the Remittent Fever - - - 77

SECT. II. Of the Cure of the Remittent Fever - - 106

CONTENTS.

Page

SECT. III. *Of the Nature and Causes of the Remittent Fever* - - 156

SECT. IV. *Of Intermittent Fevers* 206

SECT. V. *Of the Cure of Intermittent Fevers* - - 208

CHAP. IV.

Of the Dysentery - - 217

SECT. I. *Of the Symptoms of the Dysentery* - - - ib.

SECT. II. *Of the Cure of the Dysentery* - - - 223

CHAP. V.

Of the Dry-Belly-Ach - - 243

CONTENTS.

SECT. I. *Of the Symptoms of the Dry-Belly-Ach* - - 243

SECT. II. *Of the Cure of the Dry-Bell-Ach* - - - 250

SECT. III. *Of the Causes of the Dry-Belly-Ach* - - - 263

CHAP. VI.

Of Sores and Ulcers - - - 275

CHAP. VII.

Of some other Diseases to which Soldiers are subject - - 284

SECT. I. *Of the Venereal Disease* ib.

CONTENTS.

                                                Page

SECT. II. *Of some Complaints arising from Insects*   -   -   288

SECT. III. *Of Inflammatory Disorders*   -   -   -   294

SECT. IV. *Of Consumptions, Mania,
and Prickly Heat*   -   -   301

CHAP. VIII.

*Remarks on some of the Diseases of Ne-
groes*   -   -   -   305

CHAP. IX.

*Of the best Manner of taking Care
of the Sick of Armies in Jamaica,
and our other West India Islands* - 315

ERRATA.

P. 192, line 7 from the top, for *are* read *is*.
        8   —   —   *is* — *are.*

OBSERVATIONS

ON THE

DISEASES OF THE ARMY

IN JAMAICA.

INTRODUCTION.

Of the Situation, Face of the Country, Climate, and Produce of the Ifland of JAMAICA.

THE ifland of Jamaica lies in north latitude, between 17° 44′ and 18° 40′; and in longitude weft from London, between 76° and 78° 30′. It is of an oval figure, one hundred and fifty miles long from eaft to weft nearly, and about fifty miles over, where it is broadeft *.

It

* The length, breadth, and fituation of the ifland are

It is very mountainous, like most of the other West India islands. There are flat lands towards the coast almost all round the island, but they seldom extend more than a few miles into the country, and the mountains rise with a steep ascent to a great height. They are covered in most places with woods to their summits. There is a chain of them that runs from one end of the island to the other. The appearance of them is singular, their sides consisting of prominent ridges and deep gullies, formed by the immense torrents of water that rush down them, after heavy falls of rain. Their tops are commonly covered with clouds, which often hang half way down their sides, presenting a most pic-

---

are not ascertained with any tolerable degree of accuracy. There is a difference of twenty miles between the best maps that we yet have of the island. Vid. Craskell's Survey, Bellin, the West India Atlas by Jefferys, and Long's History of Jamaica.

turesque

INTRODUCTION. 3

turefque appearance. Towards the eaft end of the ifland, where they are higheft, they are called the *blue mountains*. Their height has not been afcertained by any accurate meafurement *; fome idea, however, may be formed of it, from the cold that is felt towards their top. On the fummit of the blue mountain peak, the higheft land in the ifland, the thermometer was found to range from $47°$ at fun-rife to $58°$ at noon, in the month of Auguft †.

The heat is greateft in the low lands along the fea-coaft, on the fouth fide of

---

* A geometrical meafurement, reported to have been made by Mr. M'Farlane, makes the height of the blue mountain peak 7,200 feet, or 2,400 yards, above the level of the fea. The barometrical obfervation of Dr. Clerk (Med. Comment. Edin. 1780) calculated according to General Roy's table of allowance for expanfion, gives 7,431 feet. We fhall certainly not err in faying they are above 7,000 feet high.

† Med. Comment. Edin. 1780, p. 248.

the island. The thermometer, in the months of May, June, July, August, and September, ranges from 85° to 90° between one and two o'clock of the afternoon, which is the hottest time of the day. During the other months of the year the heat is about five degrees less in the day-time; but the difference in the temperature of the nights is much more considerable: for, in the hot months, the thermometer seldom falls lower than 80° in the night-time; whereas, in December, January, February, and March, the coldest months in the year, it often descends to 70°, and I once saw it as low as 69° about sun-rise, which is the coldest time in the twenty-four hours. These observations were made in the town of Kingston *. As you ascend the mountains, the heat diminishes; at Stoney

* The thermometers used were made by Mr. Ramsden, and divided according to Fahrenheit's scale.

Hill,

Hill, which is ten miles from Kingston, and at no great height in the mountains, there is a difference of nearly ten degrees in the temperature; at Cold Spring*, the difference is not much less than 20°. In the intermediate situations there is a delightful variety of climate, which few countries can boast of; and in the small valleys, that lie among the mountains, so temperate is the air, that apples, strawberries, and other European fruits are cultivated with success, and also the same vegetables that are produced in the gardens of England.

The winds between the tropics, blow from east to west, as is well known, following the course of the sun. In the day-time they blow steadily in the island of Jamaica, making allowance for changes produced in their course

---

* Cold Spring is reputed, by Mr. M'Farlane's measurement, to be 1,400 yards above the level of the sea.

by the shape and figure of the land; but during the night, the cold air condensed on the tops of the mountains rushes down, and forms what is called the land breeze. These alternate changes greatly refresh the air, and render the heat less insupportable. In the months of November and December there are north winds, which sometimes prevail for several days together, and blow all the way from the continent of North America. They are severely felt on the north side of the island, and even pass the lofty mountains, and blow for days together on the south side.

The months of August, September, and October, are called the hurricane months, as violent storms of wind and rain happen in them. In such storms the wind does not blow in one direction, but in furious gusts, and whirlwinds from every quarter; and the weight of water giving additional force to the velocity

locity of the winds, they strip the trees of their leaves and branches, or tear them up by the roots; destroy the produce of the lands, throw down houses, and leave the country an uniform waste. It is almost incredible, what weighty and solid bodies are moved to great distances; and such examples of this are produced as would not meet with belief, were they not authenticated beyond a doubt. In the year 1780, on the 3d of October, the west end of the island was rendered almost a desart by a storm of uncommon violence, which did little or no damage in the other parts of the island. Previous to that period, Jamaica had not suffered materially from storms during the space of thirty-six years; but since that time, for six successive years, excepting the year 1782, one quarter of the island or another has been greatly injured by violent storms.

The year is divided into the dry and rainy

rainy seasons. The rains are expected in May, and October, but they are by no means regular. Of the rain that falls annually, much the greater proportion is in the six months that elapse from the middle of May to the middle of November, and that is probably not less than three quarters of the whole. The heaviest rains come from the sea, and sometimes continue incessantly one or more days, during which a prodigious quantity of water falls. The lighter showers come from the mountains, and for many days together return nearly at the same hour*. The warm winds blowing from the sea, strike against the lofty mountains; the vapour with which they are loaded is condensed into clouds, which after accumulating for some time are repelled

---

* What is here said of the rains is to be understood as applying chiefly to Kingston, and that neighbourhood. The quantity that falls annually is between 60 and 70 inches.

pelled upon the low lands, and there fall in showers. Much thunder usually accompanies this process, but it seldom does any mischief, for the high mountains appear to serve as conductors in carrying it to the earth. The high grounds seldom suffer from want of rain, though along the sea-coast the country is often parched up.

There are many rivers running in all directions from the mountains, but none navigable except Black River. They are very rapid, and when heavy rains fall in the mountains, pour down an immense torrent of water. Some of them bury themselves suddenly under ground, and after a little break out as abruptly; though there are others that cannot afterwards be traced. There are also examples of large streams of water bursting all at once from the ground; and it is probable, that among such lofty mountains, there are many subterraneous passages for water.

There

There are few places in the low lands, to which a stream of water might not be conducted; but this is not much practised as yet in the cultivation of the ground, and wells or tanks in most places supply water for domestic purposes.

The sky is rarely obscured with clouds, except during the rainy seasons; the nights are uncommonly clear, and the moon and stars shine with a brightness many degrees superior to what is seen in Europe. The rising and setting sun gilds the horizon with the most beautiful tints and colours, and exhibits a scene the most splendid in nature.

The soil, where it is not rocky *, is in general fertile. The island is well supplied with provisions of every kind, and

---

* The bare honey-comb rock, which is every where to be met with, is calcareous; and the honey-comb appearance of the surface proceeds from the air and rain acting upon, and carrying off the softer parts, while they leave the harder.

could eafily raife more than fufficient for the inhabitants; but the cultivation of the fugar-cane is fo lucrative, that every exertion is turned that way, and many articles are imported, which might either be produced in the ifland, or their room fupplied by others equally good. The beef and mutton are good, and the pork is excellent. Greens, and efculent roots of various kinds, are plentiful, and in great perfection. The tropical fruits, whereever a little care is taken of them, are fine and delicious. Along the coaft, and in the rivers, there is great variety of excellent fifh. The poultry is of the beft kind, and there is alfo plenty of wild fowl at particular feafons of the year.

CHAP. I.

Sect. I. *Of the Causes of Sickness and Mortality, among Soldiers and Europeans, in Jamaica.*

FROM the first discovery of the West Indies to the present time, all expeditions and emigrations to that part of the world have been attended with great mortality. Columbus and his companions suffered severely, and succeeding adventurers have not been more fortunate. The first military expedition of any consequence, that went from this country to the West Indies, was sent against Hispaniola by Oliver Cromwell; but failing in an attempt upon that island, they attacked Jamaica with better success. The far greater part of them in a short time perished by sickness. The unfortunate

unfortunate expedition againſt Carthagena is ſtill remembered, more from the mortality that attended it, than the want of ſucceſs: and though this country, in a ſubſequent war, was more fortunate in their attempts upon Martinique, Guadaloupe, and the Havannah, yet there were few of the conquering troops alive ſix months after their victories.

Great loſſes of a later date have been ſuſtained in the war juſt concluded, particularly at St. Lucia, Jamaica, and on the Spaniſh Main. Four regiments were ſent from England in 1780 to Jamaica; they arrived there the 1ſt of Auguſt, and before the end of January enſuing, not quite ſix months, one half of them nearly were dead, and a conſiderable part of the remainder were unfit for ſervice. Notwithſtanding theſe repeated loſſes, and the Weſt Indies having been a principal ſeat of war during the two laſt ruptures between this country and France, and being likely to become

come so again in case of another war, no steps have been taken to guard against the mortality, at least adequate to the importance of the object; and the useful experience of one war has been lost before the commencement of another. It would seem to be a proper time, at the conclusion of the present, to collect the useful lessons we have so dearly purchased, and to deduce from them the best regulations for preventing similar misfortunes in future. But the means of obtaining an object so desirable will be better understood, and may be more effectually put in execution, after some acquaintance with the usual causes of sickness, and mortality in the West Indies.

The disorders that prove fatal to soldiers, and Europeans in general in the West Indies, are of two kinds, namely fevers and fluxes. They are the concomitants of armies in all parts of the world, but in tropical climates they rage with peculiar violence.

There appears to be an intimate connection between them, for they are frequently combined together, often interchange with each other, and it rarely happens that one is epidemic without the other. They would feem to depend upon the fame caufe, perhaps differently modified. The fevers are fimilar to what have been called marfh, and remittent fevers; but greatly more violent in their attack, quicker in their progrefs, and more fatal in their termination, than what are feen in Europe. They proceed from the fame caufe, noxious exhalations from wet, low, and marfhy grounds. That fuch vapours are a caufe of fever, has been confirmed by repeated experience and obfervation, in all parts of the world.

Towards the production of fuch noxious vapours, there appears to be wanting the concurrence of three circumftances; heat, moifture, and decayed vegetable or animal matter. The heat of tropical

tropical climates, though generally reputed the cause of their unhealthiness, will not alone produce fevers, as is strongly exemplified in those living on board of ship, who remain free from fevers; and also in the inhabitants of certain dry sandy spots along the coast, in which the heat is uncommonly great, yet the situations are healthy, as Fort-Augusta, Port-Royal, and others.

Simple moisture is harmless *, at least as far as relates to the production of fevers, of which the two last-mentioned places may likewise be given as examples, for they are nearly surrounded with water on all sides. It is true, the air is perfectly clear; yet it must be loaded with moisture, in consequence of the great heat of the sun acting upon the water. But the vapour arising from water is harmless, even when rendered more

* Vid. Med. Transf. vol. ii. p. 521.

an object of our senses, by being condensed into fogs and clouds. Thus, the parish of St. Thomas's in the Vale is every night covered with a thick fog, owing to the rivers which pass through it sending forth vapours, which in the day-time are perfectly transparent; but towards evening, by the cool air coming from the neighbouring mountains, they are condensed, and remain visible till next day's sun disperse them, without however being at all unwholesome.

Dead vegetable and animal matter do not send forth noxious vapours, unless in a state of corruption, for which a certain degree both of heat and moisture is necessary. In northern climates, the heat is not sufficient till summer to raise noxious exhalations from swampy grounds; but in Jamaica such are produced all the year round from wet and marshy places, which are always found to be unhealthy, as are also those places lying to leeward of them. The dry part of the country continues healthy during the hot weather, but as foon as the rains fet in it becomes unhealthy. After heavy falls of rain, every part of the flat country feems to exhale the fame noxious vapours as marfhes; for the moifture never fails to meet with fufficient quantity of decayed vegetable or animal matter, dried and preferved by the preceding heat.

In dry fandy fpots, nearly furrounded by the fea, there is little or no decayed vegetable or animal matter; and there is no moifture, for the rain is immediately abforbed by the fand: fuch places therefore are healthy, and almoft exempt from fevers. Elevated and mountainous fituations are alfo healthy, for what there is of decayed vegetable and animal matter is wafhed away by the frequent rains, which do not penetrate the ground, but in running off carry whatever is light and loofe along with them. What is thus carried

carried off, is frequently depofited in the valleys among the hills; but thofe are fo fmall, that they do not form a bottom large enough to emit vapours hurtful in any great degree: add to this, that the inhabitants never fet down their houfes in fuch bottoms, but conftantly make choice of a lofty fituation. How much it contributes to health, being raifed even a little above the exhalations, may be judged from this, that in the flat part of the country the houfes upon a level with the ground, or but little raifed above it, are uniformly the moft unhealthy.

If any doubts be entertained, that the exhalations from wet and marfhy grounds are the caufes of fevers in Jamaica, attention to the following facts cannot fail to remove them. Ships lying at Port Royal, with their men in perfect health, on moving higher up the harbour, either oppofite to Kingfton, Rock Fort, or beyond them, and taking their ftation in any of these places, have in a few days become sickly. The men have been seized with fevers, owing to the low swampy lands along the shore, and at the head of the harbour, from which last the exhalations are carried every morning towards the ships, when the regular sea breeze sets in, as is sensibly perceived by the bad smell which accompanies it. In the year 1782, two frigates moored at the head of the harbour, to guard against an attack in that quarter, were obliged to leave their station in a fortnight, on account of sickness, though few of their people had been permitted to go on shore during that time. The ships of war do not go so high up to take in their water, but, the place being wet and swampy, it commonly happens that the men employed in filling the water casks are taken sick, either at the time, or a few days after; and there are examples where, out of sixty or seventy men on that duty, not one has escaped a fever.

In

In this particular case however, there are concurring circumstances, that give additional force to the original cause, the principal of which is intoxication from rum. This has been remarked as so pernicious, that it has become an opinion with many, that it is the principal cause of sickness in the West Indies. But there is no good ground for this, for rum does not appear to possess any specific power of producing remittent fevers or fluxes, more than other ardent or rectified spirits, which of themselves are never known to occasion those diseases*. It is further to be observed, that rum is drunk with impunity as far as regards fevers, whenever the causes abovementioned are not present, or the intoxicated person is not exposed to them. The men on board the two frigates drank as much rum while lying at Port Royal, as

* Vide Pringle, Dis. of Army. ed. 7th, p. 87.

when stationed at the top of the harbour; yet in the former situation they were perfectly healthy, and in the latter extremely sickly. The pernicious effects of rum are to be imputed to its weakening the powers of digestion in the stomach, and the constitution in general; but still more to its giving rise in a state of intoxication to excesses and irregularities, such as walking or running violently in the sun, lying down in the open air during the heat of the day or damps of the night, and going to sleep in those situations. Such things of themselves without previous intoxication, concur powerfully in rendering fevers both more violent, and more frequent.

The following particulars are likewise found to have equally pernicious effects as rum; fatigue, hard labour, bad or scanty diet, long fasting, and distress of mind of all kinds. Every thing indeed that any how weakens or exhausts the body,

body, would seem to co-operate powerfully in giving force to the original cause of fever. Exposure to rain, and thereby getting wet, are generally believed to be productive of fevers in Jamaica. All the circumstances, or the greater part of them, just mentioned, attend soldiers on actual service; and if we take into consideration the difficulty, nay often the impossibility of taking proper care of the sick in such situations, some opinion may be formed of the causes of that dreadful mortality, that has uniformly attended the armies of Europeans in the West Indies.

It is farther to be remarked, that those who are just arrived from cool and healthy climates, are particularly subject to fevers, as is daily experienced by all new comers. A regiment always loses a greater proportion of men the first year than afterwards, supposing their situation to be the same. The great and sudden

sudden heat, which renders the body feeble and languid, no doubt contributes to this; but it is chiefly to be ascribed to this circumstance, that the human frame acquires by habit a power of resisting noxious causes, as is seen every day in the use of opium, ardent spirits, and many poisonous substances. Hence Europeans, after remaining some time in the West Indies, are less liable to be affected by the causes of fevers than on their first arrival. Even in England it has been observed, that such as move from an healthy part of the country, into one that is low and full of swamps, suffer more than the original inhabitants. The negroes afford a striking example, of the power acquired by habit of resisting the causes of fevers; for, though they are not entirely exempted from them, they suffer infinitely less than Europeans. There was the strongest proof of this in the negroes who
were

were sent along with the troops against Fort *St. Juan*, of whom scarcely any died, although few or none of the soldiers survived the expedition.

It is a circumstance universally remarked, that there is a great difference in the degrees of health enjoyed by the men, and the women, in the West Indies, I mean Europeans and their descendants. The life of a woman is at least twice as good as that of a man, to speak in the terms of those, who make such things matter of calculation. This is owing to their keeping much within doors, or going out only in the cool of the morning or evening, and even then in a carriage; and to their using no violent exertions in the open air, whereby they are little exposed to the causes of fevers, against which they are further guarded by their regularity, and temperance in living. During the war there was a class of females, who had it not in their power

power to use some of the above precautions, and neglected others, that suffered as much as the men, I mean the wives of the common soldiers. The temperance of the women proving some security against fevers, it will naturally be supposed, that the intemperance of the men renders such disorders more frequent; and doubtless it is so. But an abstemious diet in men obliged to lead an active life, and to be much in the open air, is far from being a preservation against the diseases of the country: on the contrary, those who live well are observed to enjoy the best health; and it may be given as a general rule, that such as are not guilty of excess in this country, ought not to follow a stricter regimen on going to the West Indies, but rather make a small addition to their usual quantity of wine.

Sect.

SECT. II. *Of the Precautions to be taken in sending Troops to the West Indies; and of the Means of preserving their Health in that Climate.*

IN treating of the means of preserving the health and lives of soldiers, I shall mention the circumstances conducive thereto, in the order they present themselves, in sending troops from Europe to the West Indies.

I. The troops to be sent should consist of well-disciplined and not new-raised men; for the latter being less orderly, and not accustomed to the life of a soldier, suffer greatly more from the climate than men habituated to discipline, as was observable in all the young regiments sent to that part of the world. Besides, it is almost impracticable to discipline men in a country, in which they

they have so many difficulties to encounter, and where the great heat renders it impossible to exercise them in the open air, except for a short time in the morning or evening; and there is even a considerable objection against the evening exercise, which I shall have occasion to mention afterwards.

II. The men should be embarked at a proper time of the year, that is, about the month of November; in order that they may arrive in the West Indies both at the coolest, and most healthy season of the year. The inconveniencies and difficulties, necessarily accompanying a change of country, will be felt much less, if it take place at an healthy than at a sickly season. By this precaution, the troops, when intended for a garrison to any of our islands, will get accustomed to the climate before the sickly season commences. If they are designed for an expedition, it becomes of the utmost consequence

consequence that they should be dispatched from England at the proper time; and they ought to proceed directly to the place of destination, without touching at any of our islands, where they seldom fail to contract much sickness. If however it be absolutely necessary to stop at one or other of the islands, to be supplied with labouring negroes, or for other purposes that the service may require, the troops should be kept on board the transports; and the transports should be anchored in an healthy station, that is, at a distance from, and not to leeward of, marshy ground. By neglecting the above precautions, expeditions otherwise judiciously planned, have proved unsuccessful from the sickness merely and consequent mortality, with little or no opposition on the part of the enemy.

III. When the troops are embarked, which they should be on board of roomy transports, the utmost attention ought to be paid by the officers, to keep the men clean both in their perſons and berths. This is done by dividing them into two or more watches, and making them come regularly upon deck every day with their bedding; alſo by ſcraping, ſmoaking, and cleaning between decks two or three times a week, and waſhing their cloaths as often. So great improvements have been made of late years by Captain Cook, Sir John Pringle*, and others, in preſerving the health of perſons at ſea, and the knowledge of them is ſo generally diffuſed, that we ſeldom hear of ſuch mortality raging on board our ſhips as formerly: yet there are not wanting inſtances of the dreadful effects of neglecting cleanlineſs, and other precautions, even in the war juſt concluded. It is no ſmall advantage, in ſending troops to the Weſt Indies, to land them with their health

---

* Diſcourſe upon ſome late improvements of the means for preſerving the health of mariners.

unimpaired,

unimpaired, and adds greatly to their chance of living in that climate.

IV. When the troops arrive in the Weſt Indies, they ſhould be quartered in barracks erected in healthy ſituations. Whenever there is not ſufficient room in the barracks, which almoſt always happens in time of war, and houſes cannot be hired that are healthy as to ſituation, the men ſhould remain on board the tranſports, till ſome temporary buildings are erected; for the air at ſea is pure and healthy, and productive of none of the diſeaſes of the country. It has always been found moſt fatal to encamp troops in the Weſt Indies, and ſhould never be done but on actual ſervice.

In regard to healthy ſituations for barracks, there was occaſion to mention, in ſpeaking of the cauſes of ſickneſs, ſuch places as were found to enjoy particular advantages in reſpect to health.

They

They are of two kinds in Jamaica, and are most probably the same in all the other islands; namely, dry sandy peninsulas or islands near the shore, and elevated situations in the mountains. As examples of the former may be mentioned Port-Royal, and Fort-Augusta. Port-Royal has always been considered as more healthy than either Spanish-Town, or Kingston; and has accordingly been resorted to by invalids from both those places. In the years 1781 and 1782, there was a striking proof of the salubrity of the air at Fort-Augusta. A corps of loyal Americans, under the command of Lord Charles Montagu, were quartered there upwards of nine months, in which time they lost only two men, and their sick seldom amounted to twenty *.

Of elevated and mountainous situations it may be observed, that they are

* Vid. Chap. ii.

more uniformly healthy than dry and sandy places upon the coast; for the neighbourhood of marshy ground, or stagnant water, often renders these last unhealthy. From a circumstance of this kind, the troops at Fort-Augusta became subject to fevers in the year 1783. The sea rising higher than usual, overflowed the whole of the ground on which the fort stands, near a foot above the surface in some places, and on ebbing left much slime and ooze. A few days after this happened, many of the men were seized with fevers*. At no great height in the mountains, there is a considerable improvement in the salubrity of the air, which cannot be imputed to the diminution of the heat, though that renders the climate more agreeable. The station of this kind, of which the troops have had most experience, is Stoney Hill. In 1782 and 1783, the 19th and

---

* Vid. Chap. ii.

30th regiments enjoyed a degree of health there, little if at all inferior to what might have been expected in any part of England *. They seldom had more than 20 sick in hospital, and the proportion of deaths was altogether inconsiderable.

Such being the healthiness of particular situations in our West India islands, it may be matter of surprise, that the mortality should have been so great among our troops. But it is to be observed, that on actual service many of the precautions essential to health cannot be attended to, such as a proper choice of ground, and avoiding what is wet and marshy; though perhaps even in this way something might be done, if more were attempted. Whenever it is not inconsistent with the service on which soldiers are sent into that country, to keep them on board of transports, it

* Vid. Chap. ii.

would

would save the lives of thousands. Some regiments serving on board the fleet suffered very little, while others on shore were almost annihilated by the diseases of the country; so different is the air at sea from the air at land. In times of peace the health of the men kept in the islands for the support of civil government, and as a garrison for defence, has certainly not been made so much an object of attention as it deserved, considering the great importance it is of in two points of view. First, that it would save a large sum of money to the nation, expended annually in recruiting, disciplining, and conveying soldiers to the West Indies, to supply the room of those who have died: and secondly, that every step taken to preserve the lives of soldiers, may be considered as the best means of having always in that part of the world, a body of troops seasoned to the climate, and therefore of more use in case of any emergency, than double their number sent from Europe.

It will often happen in time of war, that more troops must be sent to an island than there are barracks, or accommodation for; in which case it would be advisable to send along with them from Europe, the frames of temporary wooden barracks, which might be speedily erected upon healthy spots. The expence of them would not be one third of what they would cost, if they were to be constructed in that country, where there is often both a want of materials and artificers.

V. When the troops are properly disposed of as to barracks, there should be a certain number of negroes attached to each regiment; or what perhaps would be better, a company of negroes and mulattoes should be formed in every regiment, to do whatever duty or hard work was to be done in the heat of the day, from which they do not suffer, though it would be fatal

fatal to Europeans. This regulation was adopted in part in Jamaica during the late war, and found extremely useful.

VI. The foldiers fhould be fupplied with provifions by government; for unlefs that be done, their fubfiftence will be very precarious in that country, and few things are more prejudicial to health than a fcanty and irregular diet. They fhould be divided into meffes, which fhould be infpected by an officer daily; and they fhould not be allowed to difpofe of, or exchange their provifions on any pretence, for this leads to bartering them for rum, the moft pernicious of all things.

VII. The men fhould be frequently out at exercife; and if it be in the morning, and not continued long, it will contribute to their health. The evenings are alfo cool, but there is an objection to exercifing the men at that time, which I learned from an officer of much experience in that country. Motion even the moſt moderate is attended with profuſe perſpiration, in which ſituation the men expoſing themſelves to the cool air of the night, with wet ſhirts upon their backs, become liable to colds, rheumatiſms, and other complaints. But after the morning exerciſe the heat of the day follows, and prevents any evils of that kind. It is true, ſuch might be avoided, were the men to put on dry ſhirts after the evening exerciſe; but this is ſeldom in the power of private ſoldiers, nor would it be an eaſy matter to make them take ſo much care of themſelves, if it were.

What relates to the care of hoſpitals, the ſubſiſtence of the ſick, and medical attendance, will be treated of afterwards.

CHAP. II.

Of the Number of Men loſt annually by the ſeveral Regiments in Jamaica; and of the various Degrees of Healthineſs of the different Quarters.

A SHORT review of the loſſes ſuſtained by the regiments in Jamaica, and of the various degrees of health which they enjoyed in the different quarters, will furniſh materials from which many uſeful concluſions may be deduced. It will point out the principal and aggravating cauſes of mortality, and what is of more conſequence, it will ſhew how in a great degree they may be avoided. It will beſides furniſh to a command-

commanding officer, the means of afcertaining what proportion of men will be fit for fervice at the moſt healthy, and the moſt unhealthy, feafons of the year; and alfo what diminution in their number may be expected, after a certain time.

The greateſt part of the troops were quartered at the following places; the three towns, Kingſton, Spaniſh Town, and Port Royal; the forts, Fort-Auguſta, Rock-fort, Caſtile-fort, and the barracks at the battery called the Twelve Apoſtles. There were befides barracks at Up-park, and Stoney-hill. All the abovementioned places, except Spaniſh Town and Stoney-hill, are fituated either upon, or at a fmall diſtance from, the banks of the great bafon of water that forms the harbour of Kingſton, and which with an inlet of little more than a mile, is above ten miles long, and in fome parts four or five miles broad. Spaniſh Town is fix or feven miles farther inland, and is fituated

in

in the flat and low part of the country, but without any marshes in the neighbourhood. Stoney-hill is in the mountains, about ten miles distant from Kingston, the three last of which are a steep ascent, though the road be not impassable for carriages. There are also barracks in the several parishes, but I am not in possession of facts to ascertain accurately, any thing respecting their different degrees of healthfulness; though it has always been found that a regiment, sent in small detachments to the parochial barracks, suffers greatly.

The following observations are confined to a short space of time, from the year 1779 to 1783, when the regiments were reduced to the peace establishment. I am not in possession of materials to begin the enquiry earlier than the year 1779, which is a year and an half previous to my arrival in the island.

LX

LX REGIMENT, 1ft Battalion.

Taking the regiments in the order in which they arrived in the ifland, the 1ft battalion of the 60th regiment comes firft to be confidered. It was 387 men ftrong the 1ft of February 1780; and in the courfe of the year 243 were enlifted. The proportion of deaths upon thofe two numbers added together, rather exceeded 3-11ths of the whole; and of difcharged men the proportion was rather more than 1-9th. The lofs to the fervice in both was nearly 2-5ths of the whole, in the courfe of one year. The regiment was quartered at Spanifh Town, had been already fome time in the ifland, and might be confidered as feafoned. The great mortality proceeded from a detachment of nearly 200 men, who were fent upon the expedition againft Fort St. Juan, of whom few or none ever returned.

The fecond year, the deaths were rather more

more than 1-6th, and the discharged did not quite amount to that number: the loss to the service in both was about 1-3d; and was in part still to be ascribed to the detachment sent on the expedition against Fort St. Juan. In the course of the year, the proportion of sick varied from 1-6th to 1-13th of the whole nearly. They were never more than the first-mentioned number, nor less than the last. Under the denomination of sick are included not merely those in the hospital, but also convalescents, and all such who from slight ailments were unable to do duty.

The third year, the deaths were about 1-8th, the discharged nearly 1-4th; and the loss in both about 3-8ths. It was six months from the conclusion of the third year, to the time of the regiment being reduced to the peace establishment, and taking the proportion upon those six months, and the preceding six months, which make the last year, they are nearly the same; that is, the deaths are between

1-8th

1-8th and 1-9th, and the discharged are above 1-4th. The great number discharged, was owing to the recruits being bad that were sent from England, which must unavoidably be the case towards the end of a war; and was also preparatory to a reduction of the regiment to the peace establishment. The sick varied from 1-5th to 1-18th during the third year; and from 1-5th to 1-24th during the last.

From the last returns it will appear, that Spanish Town may be considered as not an unhealthy quarter for soldiers. The deaths are in the proportion of one to eight, and it is computed that one in ten of the inhabitants dies annually. The difference of mortality in the first and last years, is in part to be imputed to the hospitals being better supplied with proper diet for the sick, and the medical attendance being more regular and frequent.

The loss to the service, the first year that

the several REGIMENTS. 45

that a regiment is in the island, is almost all by deaths. The second year the deaths are considerably diminished, but the number of those who are enfeebled, or worn out by disease is increased, and therefore the discharged men form a large part of those who are lost to the service.

The sickly months are always determined by the fall of the rains. The mortality is not greatest at the most sickly time of the year, but about one or two months after, when the men that have been worn out by repeated attacks of fever, can no longer withstand the disease. Hence the greatest number of deaths are in October and November, though the sick are generally most numerous in August and September.

LXXIX REGIMENT.

The 79th regiment arrived in Jamaica in July 1779, 1,008 men strong. They were quartered in Kingston. The first year they lost nearly 2-7ths by death. The second

second year they lost 4-7ths by death, but 300 of those were men sent upon the expedition against Fort St. Juan; setting aside therefore that number, and taking the proportion upon the remainder, the deaths were nearly 5-18ths, which is not much less than that of the preceding year. The discharged men the second year were 1-6th; and the loss to the service, including both dead and discharged, 4-9ths nearly. This great mortality was, among other causes, to be imputed to an unhealthy quarter. The proportion of sick, during the second year, varied from 1-half nearly to 1-5th of the whole.

The third year the regiment was very weak. There died 1-11th; there were discharged 1-8th; and the loss in both was nearly 3-14ths. The sick varied from 2-7ths to 1-6th.

The fourth year, the regiment was reinforced by men drafted from the regiments, that were sent home. They lost 1-4th by death, and 1-6th were discharged: in both the lofs amounted to 5-12ths. The fick varied from 1-half to 1-5th. So great a difference in the mortality of this and the preceding year, while the obvious difference in the ftate of the regiment in the two years was, that in the firft they were weak, and in the fecond ftrong, leads to a fufpicion that the accommodation, number of officers, and other circumftances, were equal to the care of 350, but not of 700 men.

In four years there died 910 men, including thofe that were loft upon the expedition againft Fort St. Juan; there were difcharged in the fame time above 200; and the lofs in both exceeded their original number by 100.

LXXXVIII REGIMENT.

The 88th regiment arrived in Jamaica, in March 1780, complete from England. In the firft year there died about 1-3d. In the fecond year the deaths were nearly 1-5th, and the difcharged 1-7th; and the

the lofs in both about 1-3d. The fick varied the firft year from 1-3d to 1-5th; in the fecond from 3-7ths to 1-6th. The regiment remained four months in the ifland after the conclufion of the fecond year, till they were drafted, and in that time loft by death 1-11th, and by difcharged men 1-12th.

During two years and four months there died about 7-16ths; and including difcharged men the lofs to the fervice was 550 out of 791, which laft number comprehends the original ftrength of the regiment, and alfo the enlifted men.

The great mortality in the regiment during the firft year, was owing to their being quartered at Rock and Caftile forts, two moft unhealthy ftations. After remaining there fome time they were removed to Fort-Augufta, but a detachment was left at their old quarters, which added greatly to the fick lift, and to the mortality. It is alfo to be obferved, that this was a new-raifed regiment.

ment. The loss the first year was nearly all by death; the second year half the loss was in discharged men.

Taking the proportions for the last twelve months, during which the principal part of the regiment was at Kingston, and a detachment at Port-Royal part of the time, there died 1-5th, there were discharged 1-7th, and the loss to the service was about 1-3d. From a comparison of the returns of the 60th regiment, and those of the two last regiments, Kingston appears to be a much less healthy quarter than Spanish Town.

The 85th, 92d, 93d, and 94th regiments were embarked at Plymouth nearly at the same time, and they all arrived in Jamaica about the end of July or beginning of August 1780. They were new-raised regiments, and from the time of their embarkation to their being landed in Jamaica, there had elapsed about six months. They arrived at the most unhealthy time of the year, and there were no quarters for their reception, nor suitable hospitals for the sick. The mortality, from all these circumstances combining with the climate, was unusually great.

LXXXV REGIMENT.

The 85th regiment were encamped in part, and quartered in part at Rock-Fort, for a short time; they were afterwards placed in barracks built at Up-Park. It should be observed, that the regiment lost few men while on board the transports, owing to the great attention that was paid to cleanliness; yet they arrived sickly, and many were scorbutic after being so long at sea. There died in the first year 5-12ths; and the loss to the service, including the discharged men, was altogether nearly 1-half. The sick varied from 1-half to 2-9ths of the whole.

In the second year, or rather the next eleven months, for before the year was completed the regiment was drafted, the proportion of deaths was rather more than 1-8th, and of discharged men 1-14th: the loss in both was nearly 1-5th. The sick varied from 1-3d to 1-8th.

The difference between this and the preceding year, is to be imputed to the regiment being seasoned, to their being lodged in good barracks, and to proper provision being made for taking care of the sick.

It may be laid down as a maxim, that no troops can stand encampment, even for a few weeks, in the low and flat parts of the West India Islands.

The quarters at Up-Park are scarcely more healthy than those at Kingston.

One cause of sickness in this regiment deserves to be taken notice of, as the other regiments were also exposed to it in their turn, that is, the duty of the prison guard. There were a great many prisoners brought to Jamaica at different times by the ships of war, and the place in which they were confined necessarily required a guard. The prison was at the distance of two miles from the quarters of the 85th regiment, and was low as to situation, being close upon the shore. It was found that a large proportion of the soldiers, sent on this duty, were seized with fevers.

XCII REGIMENT.

The 92d regiment were quartered at Spanish Town; they were ill supplied with every necessary for their hospital, and they were much confined in their quarters. In the first year there died nearly 5-12ths; there were discharged 1-25th; and the loss in both was about 11-25ths. The sick varied from 1-half, or rather more, to 1-28th.

The second year, or more properly the

the next eleven months, the deaths were not quite 1-12th; and the difcharged men were 1-14th: the lofs in both was between 1-6th and 1-7th. The fick varied from 1-12th to 1-38th. This is a fuperior degree of health to that enjoyed by the 85th regiment at Up-Park; and though there may have been other circumftances that contributed to it, yet it no doubt depended principally on the quarters at Spanifh Town being more healthy than thofe at Up-Park, as farther appeared, by the number of fick admitted into the hofpitals being much greater in the latter, than in the former place.

When the 85th and 92d regiments were drafted, in the former there were 219 men fit for fervice; in the latter there were 277. The 85th regiment had enlifted 148, the 92d regiment 41; and they both arrived in the ifland nearly 600 men ftrong. Of the 85th regiment there remained of the original number 71, at the end of one year and eleven months from their arrival in the island; of the 92d regiment there remained 236. It is to be observed, that the last-mentioned regiment were sickly when they arrived in Jamaica, owing to their having been so long on board the transports; but they lost few or none on the passage, from the attention that was paid to keep the men, and ships clean.

XCIII REGIMENT.

The 93d regiment were quartered at Kingston. They were sickly on board the transports, and many died on the passage. They landed a great number sick, and in all they amounted to 404 men. In the space of six months upwards of 1-half died; and of the remainder only 71 were fit for service, who were drafted into another regiment. At the end of six months the loss to the service, in dead and discharged, amounted to 9-11ths of the original number.

The

The causes of a mortality so dreadful, are to be found in their being new-raised and undisciplined men, sickly and scorbutic on board the transports, arriving in the island at the most unhealthy time of the year, being in bad quarters, and having no adequate provision for the great number of sick.

XCIV REGIMENT.

The 94th regiment were very sickly on board the transports, and lost some men on the passage. They landed 531 men, and were immediately sent in small detachments to the different country quarters. By the end of the first year there were upwards of 1-half dead. In the second year there died 2-7ths of the remainder. At the end of two years and four months, there remained of the whole number 1-7th fit for service, who were drafted into another regiment. Thus, the loss to the service was 6-7ths of the whole in two years and four months.

In the above four regiments there died, in the firſt ſix months, rather more than 2-5ths of the numbers landed.

It is with horror, that we thus ſee our fellow-creatures ſacrificed in thouſands to the dreadful viciſſitudes of climate, combined with other cauſes of mortality: and if ſuch be the caſe in our own iſlands, where there are no enemies to encounter, and where the evils of the climate are not aggravated by the fatigues and hardſhips unavoidably attending actual ſervice, ſome idea may be formed of the dreadful havock, that muſt enſue among European troops, when thoſe cauſes are combined.

The firſt expedition of any note, ſent from this country to the Weſt Indies, was that againſt Hiſpaniola under Cromwell. They failed in their attempt upon that iſland, but afterwards attacked Jamaica,

Jamaica, where they met with little refiftance. There were above 10,000 land forces fent upon the expedition, yet we find them calling for reinforcements, almoft as foon as they were in poffeffion of the ifland; and in a fhort time after, reprefenting the difadvantages arifing from fending new-raifed men*.

In the unfuccefsful expedition againft Carthagena, of the troops landed, and who remained on fhore only ten days, the lofs in that time was one fourth of the whole nearly, of whom by much the greater part fell a facrifice to the climate. When they were embarked, the number of fick, compared with thofe that were well, was in the proportion of 2 to 5.

The dreadful mortalities attending the fuccefsful expeditions againft Martinique, Guadaloupe, and the Havannah, are ftill frefh in the memories of many. It is fufficient to fay, that a very fmall part of

* Letters in the public offices, Jamaica.

the victorious troops were alive, three months after their conquests.

In the late war, 5,000 of the bravest troops in the world took possession of the island of St. Lucia: their loss in killed and wounded, in the several unequal and desperate attacks that were made upon them by the enemy, was not considerable; but at the end of a twelvemonth, scarcely a man remained of the original number. The mortality continued as great in the subsequent years. From the 1st of May 1780 to the 1st of May 1781, the number of dead was equal to the average strength of the garrison during the year. Of the troops sent upon the expedition against Fort St. Juan from Jamaica, scarcely a man ever returned.

The mind recoils with horror, from such scenes of destruction of the human species; and in returning more immediately to the subject of the health of the regiments in Jamaica, there is this consolation, folation, that no examples of mortality occur equal to thofe already mentioned; and that the facts to be ftated fuggeft the means, whereby a remedy may be provided againſt ſo great an evil.

DUKE OF CUMBERLAND's REGIMENT.

The Duke of Cumberland's regiment, a provincial corps raiſed in America, and confifting of native Americans from the fouthern provinces, arrived in Jamaica in 1781. They were quartered in Fort-Augufta, and remained there nine months; in which time the deaths were 1-52th. Only one man was difcharged, and the fick varied from 1-12th to 1-30th. Soldiers cannot be expected to enjoy better health in any country; and it was fufpected, that having been uſed to heats not inferior to thofe of tropical climates, they were lefs liable to the difeaſes of the Weſt Indies. But there was no good ground for this fuppofition, as appeared on the regiment being moved from Fort Augusta, which happened in the end of April. They went to Stoney Hill, and remained there four months, in which time six men died, and four were discharged. The proportions taken for the thirteen months were in deaths 2-67ths; in discharged 1-108th; and the loss in both 1-26th, which for the year is not a loss of more than 1-28th.

The next year they were quartered at Kingston; there died rather more than 2-13ths; there were discharged 1-60th; and the loss in both was 4-23ths, that is, more than 1-6th. The sick varied from 1-7th to nearly 1-half of the whole. The mortality though great, is still less than what other regiments suffered in the same quarters, which is to be imputed to two causes; first, that the men were in part seasoned to the climate; and secondly, that the Americans were more orderly, and less guilty of excess in drinking,

drinking, than the British soldiers. The greatest mortality happened in the months of November and December, though the sick were most numerous in the preceding months.

XIV REGIMENT.

The 14th regiment arrived in Jamaica in April 1782. Five companies were quartered at Spanish Town, and five at Fort Augusta; and these last, after three months, were moved to Spanish Town, where the whole regiment remained. In the first year there died 1-6th nearly, and 1-10th were discharged *; the loss to the service in both was 4-15ths, or more than a quarter. This regiment enjoyed

---

* This number of discharged men is greater than common for the first year, which is to be imputed to the regiment having been in Hilsey barracks previous to their embarkation, whereby many of the men had their health greatly injured, by the fevers produced by that unhealthy quarter.

most of the advantages that troops can have, that are sent to Jamaica. It was an old regiment, in good order, and they arrived at an healthy time of the year. The quarters they were put into at Spanish Town, may be considered as a mean between the most, and the least, healthy. The sick were well provided with hospitals, provisions, and attendance; and their numbers varied from 1-7th to 2-7ths of the whole. Notwithstanding all these advantages the mortality is great, yet inconsiderable when compared with the numbers lost by the 92d regiment in the same quarters, during their first year. The deaths of the one were 5-12ths, and of the other only 1-6th. There is a circumstance that should be taken notice of here, as it sets in a proper light the degree of healthiness of the quarters at Spanish Town: a large proportion of the sick and of the deaths, both in the 14th regiment, and in the 1st battalion of the 60th

60th regiment, during the laft year, was owing to an out-poft, eight or nine miles diftant from Spanifh Town, to which the two regiments fent detachments. The detachments were fmall, but in general almoft all the men fent upon that duty were brought to the hofpital, and many of them with fevers of the worft kind.

In the fame quarters, the 14th regiment loft by deaths 1-6th, and the 60th regiment 1-8th; which difference is to be imputed to the latter being feafoned. It is to be taken into the account, that the 60th regiment had a confiderable number of recruits fent from England, which increafed the mortality. The 92d regiment, in the fame quarters, during the fecond year loft nearly 1-11th: it may not therefore be unfair to conclude, that in fimilar circumftances, the mortality will be nearly twice as great the firft year as the fecond.

XIX

XIX and XXX REGIMENTS.

Seven companies of the 19th and 30th regiments arrived in Jamaica in July 1782; and were quartered at Stoney Hill. In the six following months, which include the sickly season, they lost by deaths 1-26th.

The remainder of the 19th regiment arrived in January 1783, and were placed in the same quarters, where they remained eight months longer, till the regiment was reduced to the peace establishment; and in that time there died 1-27th.

The remaining companies of the 30th regiment, arrived at the same time with those of the 19th regiment, and were quartered also eight months longer at Stoney Hill, in which time there died 1-34th. The annual mean of deaths upon the whole was 1-17th nearly.

The discharged men in the first six months, were 1-94th from the seven companies; during the following eight months, they were 1-19th from the 19th regiment; and 1-32d from the 30th regiment : the annual average of discharged men upon these is 1-21th nearly. Taking therefore the loss by death and discharged men together, it is somewhat more than 1-10th. Small as this loss must appear, when compared with the mortalities before mentioned, there are several circumstances that deserve to be taken notice of, which give a still more favourable idea of the healthiness of this quarter. The whole number of dead in the returns, did not actually die at Stoney Hill; several of them died before the two regiments joined those companies, that first arrived. The number of the dead in the surgeon's returns on the spot, do not much exceed the half of those in the general return, which included those that died

died at Jamaica, as well as elsewhere. Of those that died at Stoney Hill, several were taken ill either at Kingston, where they were upon leave, or on the road back to the barracks.

The 19th and 30th regiments were not seasoned to the climate, and they arrived at a sickly time of the year, yet their loss was greatly less than that of the regiments at Spanish Town that were seasoned, and where every possible care was taken both of the men that were well, and of the sick. Such are the superior advantages of the quarters at Stoney Hill. The sick varied from 1-6th to 1-10th, but most of them were trifling sores that were not taken into the hospital. The sick in hospital varied from 1-22th to 1-36th only.

XCIX REGIMENT.

The 99th regiment was very unfortunate, being nearly all captured on their passage

passage to Jamaica. About three companies arrived in 1781, which were sent into country quarters, and the regiment did not assume any form till July 1782, when they were collected all together at Fort Augusta. They remained there several months, and sent detachments to Port-Royal, and the Twelve Apostles; a considerable number were also embarked on board the men of war, to serve as marines; and they were afterwards quartered on the *Pallisades,* where temporary barracks were erected. The name of *Pallisades* is given to a long sand-bank, which separates the harbour of Kingston from the sea. The situation is of the same kind as that of Fort-Augusta. In the year they lost by deaths 1-11th; by discharged men 2-11ths; and by both 3-11ths. This loss may be considered as great, as they were in healthy quarters; but the men collected from the parochial barracks were sickly and worn out, and increased both the number of dead and discharged, but particularly the last; add to this, the recruits that composed one half of the regiment were not good men, as must be the case towards the end of a war.

III, LXIII, LXIV, and LXXI REGIMENTS.

These regiments, or rather the remains of them, arrived from Charlestown, South Carolina, in January 1783: they amounted in all to about 800 men.

The 3d and 63d regiments were quartered at Fort-Augusta. In eight months there died of the 3d 1-23d. They arrived sickly, and many of the men were worn out by the fevers, under which they had laboured in South Carolina. The sick varied from 1-5th to 1-29th; they arrived with the former number, and when they left the fort they had nearly the same proportion, in consequence of the sea rising

to

the several REGIMENTS.

to an unusual height, overflowing the fort, and leaving stagnant water to putrefy, which produced many fevers both in this regiment, and in the 63d.

The 63d regiment arrived sickly; they had 2-7ths on the sick list. The deaths in eight months were 1-10th nearly. The sick after a short time fell to 1-13th, and did not exceed that number, till raised by the inundations above mentioned.

The 64th regiment was quartered at Port-Royal, and in eight months time lost by deaths 1-123th. The sick varied from 1-8th to 1-16th. Port-Royal stands upon a bank of sand, in the same way that Fort-Augusta does, and is a healthy quarter; it would be more so, if the town were kept cleaner, and if there were fewer shops in it, that retailed spirituous liquors.

The 71st regiment was quartered at the Twelve Apostles, which is situated upon a rock, and is also an healthy quarter.

ter. In eight months the deaths were 1-65th; and the sick varied from 2-9ths to 1-7th.

AN average of the number of sick during three years and an half, in which are included the convalescents, gives 1-3d of the army unfit for service, at the time of the greatest sickness, and 1-8th, at the time of the least sickness. The average of deaths annually upon the whole, is nearly one in four, and of discharged men about one in eight, which together make the loss 3-8ths of the whole.

In less than four years, there died in the island of Jamaica 3,500 men; those that were discharged amounted to one half of that number, which make in all 5,250

5,250 men, loft to the fervice in that fhort period of time, from the climate and other caufes of mortality, without a man dying by the hands of the enemy.

The mifchievous effects of fending new-raifed men to the Weft Indies, are exemplified in the ftrongeft manner, in all the young regiments. The mortality has likewife been greatly increafed on many occafions, by the troops leaving England at an improper feafon, and arriving in the Weft Indies at the fickly time of the year. But what has the greateft influence, of all the circumftances that affect the health of foldiers in thofe climates, is the kind of quarters in which they are placed. Kingfton and Up-Park are both bad quarters; and Rock-Fort, from the fwampy ground in its neighbourhood, and on which it ftands, is ftill worfe. Spanifh Town is better than Kingfton, though greatly inferior to Fort-Augufta or Stoney-Hill; indeed thefe two laft quarters would not be reckoned unhealthy, in any part of the world. Similar situations are to be found in all parts of Jamaica, and, I doubt not, in most, if not all, of the other West India islands. The situations are of two kinds; dry sand-banks, surrounded either wholly, or in part, by the sea, and out of the reach of noxious winds blowing from swamps and marshes; and elevated stations in the mountains. In places so circumstanced, the effects of the remittent fever are scarcely felt.

If we may be allowed to make the supposition, that quarters had been provided for the troops in such situations, of 5,250 men lost to the service, there would have remained, at the end of three years and an half, 3,500 fit for duty, supposing them to have been placed at Stoney-Hill, and to have suffered the greatest losses that have happened in that quarter.

No attendance or care of the sick can counterbalance

counterbalance the ill effects, arising from the quarters in which the troops have hitherto been placed. By professional skill, and diligence, the life of the individual may often indeed be preserved, but the *soldier* is lost to his country: and the national purposes, for which he is conveyed into those distant provinces, are as effectually frustrated by the ruin of his health, as they would be by his death. Our humanity alone is not interested in the present case, though surely the object well deserves that it should; but the safety of the West Indies, and the saving of enormous sums to government. If the troops, sent for the defence of our islands, die as we have seen them, the mother country cannot long supply, during a war, such an incessant drain: besides, the mortality is sometimes so great and speedy, that a sufficient interval is not left to make known the want of men, and receive supplies in proper time. In April 1782,

1782, when Jamaica was expected to be attacked, though upwards of 7,000 men had been sent there in the three preceding years, there were not above 2,000 men fit for duty.

It may be permitted to point out another advantage, and not an inconsiderable one, that would result from placing the troops in the healthy quarters mentioned above. The nation would at all times have a body of seasoned men in the West Indies, which in military operations either offensive or defensive, in that quarter of the world, would be of more value than twice the number of the best troops, that could be sent from Europe. Such an object must be of consequence, as the West Indies have been a principal scene of action in the two last wars, and are likely to become so again in any subsequent war.

To conclude, the interest of government, the safety of our West India possessions,

sessions, and the calls of humanity, are all equally concerned, in providing quarters for the troops in healthy situations. That such are to be found in the island of Jamaica, is proved by full and repeated experience; and there is this farther to be said in their recommendation, that they are in general favourably circumstanced for the defence of the country. Stoney Hill, of which mention has so often been made, was deemed by Sir John Dalling, and Sir Archibald Campbell, both officers highly distinguished for their military knowledge, a most advantageous post for the defence of the island.

CHAP.

CHAP. III.

Of Fevers.

THE fevers, that prevail in Jamaica, are either of the intermittent, or remittent kind. Of the former there are tertians, quartans, and quotidians, in all the various forms they occasionally assume. The remittent fevers are both the most frequent, and most fatal. There appears to be an intimate connection between them; the intermittent often running into the remittent; and the remittent sometimes terminating in an intermittent. It would seem that they proceeded from the same cause, acting with more or less violence at different times; for, in the

the more healthy feafon of the year, the fevers are chiefly intermittent, and in the moft unhealthy, remittent.

Sect. I. *Of the Symptoms of the Remittent Fever.*

PERSONS at all times of life, from infancy to old age, are fubject to the remittent fever. It attacks, however, men oftener than women; and young children, till they reach their third or fourth year, are not fo liable to it as afterwards; old people are likewife lefs fubject to it. This, probably, is not owing fo much to there being any thing either in age or fex that refifts the fever, as to perfons of the above defcription being lefs expofed to the caufes of it.

It

It is both moſt violent and moſt fatal, in thoſe who are lately arrived in the iſland, and they are at their firſt coming more ſubject to it than afterwards.

The uſual manner in which it ſhews itſelf is as follows. There is uneaſineſs with languor, followed by a ſenſe of chillineſs or cold ſhiverings, which are ſoon ſucceeded by great heat, particularly in the palms of the hands and forehead; head-ach, great loſs of ſtrength, ſickneſs at ſtomach, and frequently violent vomiting. Phlegm, or what was eaten at the laſt meal unchanged, is firſt brought up, and afterwards bile, yellow, or greeniſh. The pulſe is quick, and at firſt ſmall; it ſoon becomes full but is ſeldom hard. There is not unfrequently much pain in the ſmall of the back, or a ſenſe of foreneſs in ſome of the limbs, which is ſometimes diffuſed all over the body, as if it had been beaten and bruiſed. Reſtleſsneſs, great anxiety, oppreſſion at the breaſt, breaft, and frequent fighings, are common fymptoms, and fometimes rife to fuch an height, that the fick appear to labour greatly in their breathing. There is not however any difficulty in diftinguifhing thofe fymptoms, from laborious refpiration, that depends upon a local affection of the lungs. In the latter the difficulty of breathing is uniform, whereas in the former both the expirations and infpirations will for two or three times together be natural and eafy, and immediately after become laborious and unequal, and fo on alternately. The vomiting is at times conftant and violent, efpecially in the worft kinds of the difeafe; and the blood being frequently in a diffolved ftate, is forced into the ftomach, and thrown up, forming what has been called by the Spaniards the *black vomit*. The blood is faid fometimes to tinge the urine and faliva, and even to iffue from the pores of the fkin; none of which

appearances

appearances I have ever feen; though in the moſt unhealthy parts of tropical climates, when difeafes are aggravated by the fatigue and hardſhips attending troops on actual fervice, they are reported to occur, and not unfrequently. As the heat increafes the face gets fluſhed, the fenfes are more affected, and the patient often becomes either wild and delirious, or drowfy and lethargic. Thefe fymptoms, after a time, are fucceeded by a fweat, which is often profufe, and gradually procures an abatement of the fever.

The length of the fit varies confiderably. It fometimes terminates in fix or feven hours, though its duration is more commonly from fifteen to twenty-four hours. In fome inſtances it extends even to thirty-fix and forty-eight hours; and I. faw one example of it continuing three complete days, without any marks of remiffion. The feveral ſtages of the

fit,

fit, known under the names of, the cold, the hot, and the fweating, vary likewife confiderably in their duration. The cold ftage is generally very flight, and often there is none at all, which I believe in fome meafure is owing to the heat of the climate; for, I obferved that the rigors and fhiverings were more confiderable in the cold, than in the hot months. I have, however, in a few inftances, feen the cold fit laft above half an hour, with fevere rigors all over the body. The hot ftage conftitutes by much the longeft part of the paroxyfm, and is generally terminated by a fweat. This is not however always the cafe, for the fever fometimes remits gradually, without any fenfible increafe in the perfpiration: nor is every fweat that occurs during the hot fit, even though profufe, critical as to a remiffion; for, a great perfpiration will fometimes continue one or more hours, and go off without at all relieving the fymptoms.

The tongue is at firſt white, and if the fever be violent, and conſiſt of two or three fits, it grows brown and dry, and even becomes chopt. The thirſt is commonly great, though in ſome caſes it is not increaſed. The urine is little changed by the fever, being always high-coloured in warm climates. With the fluſhing of the face, the eye often becomes muddy, and even red, as if enflamed; and this appearance keeps pace with the progreſs of the fever, the redneſs being greateſt when the fever is higheſt, and gradually decreaſing as the remiſſion takes place.

Hitherto the difference between the fever of this iſland, and thoſe occurring in other countries, is not very conſiderable; but the ſeverity of the ſymptoms, as a ſudden and almoſt entire loſs of ſtrength, a great degree of ſtupor and even total inſenſibility, followed by convulſive ſtartings of the tendons and death, mark an extreme degree of violence,

lence, and are rarely obferved in the fevers of other countries at fo early a period; for, all thofe will fometimes happen during the firft paroxyfm, and even in the fpace of twelve hours. One of the more violent fymptoms, which frequently occurs, is inceffant retching or vomiting, with great pain at the pit of the ftomach. It not only harraffes and weakens the patient, but by preventing the ufe of any medicine, either for the immediate relief of the fever, or to prevent a return, is attended with imminent danger.

The remiffions vary much in their duration; fome do not laft longer than one or two hours, though more commonly they continue ten or fifteen, and fometimes thirty, and even thirty-fix hours. The fever in fome cafes affumes the quotidian type, and has an exacerbation every day at nearly the fame hour; but generally it obferves no regularity in the times, either of accefs, or remiffion. The remissions are more or less complete; sometimes they amount almost to an intermission, though much more generally there is only an abatement of the symptoms. The pulse becomes slower, the skin cooler, and the head-ach, restlessness, and sickness diminish, or go entirely off. Yet it sometimes happens that the remission is not so strongly marked, and is only to be distinguished by an abatement of the head-ach and restlessness, with some diminution of the quickness of the pulse, and of the heat of the skin. In judging of the heat of the skin, the feel of the sick person's hand is not to be trusted to; for, the perspiration rising freely in vapour from every pore, gives a coolness to the hand, which would lead to an erroneous opinion. The feel of the cheek, and particularly the forehead, is what best marks the degree of febrile heat.

The sleep, during the remission, is disturbed, and procures but little refreshment.

The second fit is always more severe than the first, if nothing has been done to check the progress of the fever. It is commonly without any cold stage, or even sense of chilliness. All the symptoms run higher; the skin is hotter, the pulse quicker, the head-ach greater, the senses more confused, the thirst often intense, and a *delirium* or *coma* come on more quickly and with greater violence, and sometimes terminate in convulsions and death.

As the delirium approaches, the eyes look wild, the voice becomes quick, and it changes from the natural tone to a sharper; there is also extreme eagerness in every motion, with an incessant tumbling, and change of posture. Wild imaginations of threatened danger, or of important business demanding immediate execution, soon follow; and in consequence of them, efforts often extremely violent, either to repel the danger, or accomplish the fancied business.

business. In attempting this they become outrageous, tremble all over, and are shook with frequent convulsive startings. From this state of excessive irritation, in which the recollection of persons and of things is equally confounded, the sick gradually sink into a kind of *stupor*. Articulation becomes difficult, the voice faulters, and instead of speech there is only a muttering; they cannot be roused to give an answer, and the tremors and startings still continue. With all these symptoms, and the pulse beating 128 in a minute, the fever will sometimes remit, the patient recover his senses, and if advantage be taken of the remission, life may often be preserved.

The sick sometimes sink into a lethargic state, without any previous delirium. They are roused with difficulty, and can only give an answer to the simplest questions, after which they immediately fall again into a state of insensibility. They can

can give no account of their feelings, or of the manner in which they were feized, and in general have not the fmalleft recollection, not even as of a dream, of any perfon or thing, that has been before them, while in that fituation.

It is however to be obferved, that though both the delirious and comatofe ftate are frequent occurrences, they are not effential to the fever, which often exifts in all its violence, and proves quickly fatal, without the fenfes being materially affected. There is indeed a way, in which the fever terminates fatally, that is often not at all fufpected. The violence of the fit begins gradually to abate, the fkin grows cooler, the pulfe flower, and the fenfes, if difordered, become more clear and diftinct. Thefe are flattering fymptoms, and in fuch a fituation danger is fcarcely apprehended; yet, if the ftrength be gone, if the countenance be languid and funk, if there be a

total

total indifference to food or nourishment, even though not rejected, and an aversion to every exertion even the smallest either of the mind or body, and if the pulse at the same time that it becomes slower is also weaker, though the patient complain of nothing, he is fast approaching to his end, and dies in a few hours; his pulse all the time indicating no danger, till excited by the pangs of death. When the recollection is tolerably distinct, which it often is, the patient is frequently the first to give notice of the approaching danger, from certain sensations of internal weakness which he feels. When such a termination happens, it is commonly after the second or third fit, particularly when the disease is very violent, and affects those, who are lately arrived in the island.

When the fever is thus severe, a symptom often occurs, which has given a name to the disease, as if a distinct one; I mean a yellow-a yellowneſs of the eyes and ſkin, from which it has been called the *yellow-fever*. This happens chiefly to new-comers, their fevers being the worſt; but it is not confined to them, for it appears ſometimes in the natives, and in thoſe who have reſided ſeveral years in the iſland. It is produced by the addition of a jaundice to the other ſymptoms of the fever. I call it jaundice, becauſe in no reſpect did the yellowneſs appear to differ from that, which uſually accompanies that diſeaſe. It is firſt to be obſerved in the eyes, and next tinges the neck and ſhoulders, and afterwards the whole body. The urine is alſo of a very deep colour, and ſtains linen rag yellow, like to that of a perſon in the jaundice. There appeared no reaſon for ſuſpecting a diſſolution of the blood to be the cauſe of the yellowneſs, for it happened frequently when no marks of ſuch diſſolution were to be found; and when they were preſent, they were not neceſſarily accompanied

panied with a yellowness of the skin. They never indeed occurred to me together, from which I would not infer that they never are combined, but only that they are not connected as cause and effect. The fever was always violent, and generally attended with pain at the pit of the stomach and severe retchings. It was characterised by the usual exacerbations and remissions, and had no peculiar symptom, except the yellowness, to intitle it to be considered as a distinct disease.

This change of colour in the skin, though most common in the fevers of the West Indies, is not confined to them, being frequently observed in other warm climates. There are instances of jaundice accompanying the fits of intermittent fevers in England, and I have seen two examples of yellowness, or jaundice in the hospital or jail fever*.

* Haller, *Opera Minora*, vol. III. p. 374, describes an epidemic fever in which the body turned yellow.

the REMITTENT Fever.

The yellowness in the yellow fever appears sometimes towards the end of the first fit, though more commonly after the second or third; and the unexpected and fatal termination of the fever, mentioned above, happens both when this symptom is present, and when it is not. I will not attempt to give any explanation of it at present, meaning to confine myself to a plain narration of facts, and to reserve for another place whatever relates to matter of opinion, and conjecture.

If the patient should survive even a third or a fourth fit, he remains almost totally deprived of strength, and frequently has still other evils awaiting him, as an attack of dysentery, which often proves fatal to such as have been previously reduced by the fever. It ought indeed to be observed, that it is no uncommon thing for the bowels to be affected with griping or purging, accompanied with dysenteric stools, during the fever.

fever. This combination of dyfentery and fever would feem to depend upon fomething in the feafon, for in one year it fhall be very common, and not fo in another. At all times, however, the fever if neglected, or ill treated, is apt to terminate in dyfentery, efpecially in foldiers.

Convalefcents are fubject to relapfes, which happen often in this fever, and are no lefs dangerous than the firft attack. They are moft frequent during the fickly feafon, and are readily produced by fatigue, expofure to the heat of the fun, or any irregularity. Sometimes they recur at various intervals, as fix or feven days, fifteen or fixteen, or twenty-five and thirty days; and this for a long time together, but without any great exactnefs in their periods; and each return commonly confifts of one, two, or more fits of the fever. Under fuch circumftances the difeafe often produces dropfy,

with

the REMITTENT *Fever.* 93

with enlargements and indurations of the liver and spleen, which in many instances terminate in death.

The violence of the symptoms, and degree of danger, such as above described, take place chiefly, in those who are but lately arrived in tropical climates, and during the most sickly season of the year. In the natives, and those who have resided some time in the island, the fever is by no means so formidable, being neither so violent in its onset, nor so rapid in its progress. It often begins in slight feverish fits, one or two of which shall pass, and the patient pay little regard to them; yet a third or fourth shall not be much short of the violence of symptoms already described. It sometimes begins as a regular intermittent, which is changed into a remittent, the fits gradually getting worse, and running into one another.

Though the fever be more gradual in its approaches in the natives and
old

old inhabitants, yet when it rifes to a great height, they are longer in recovering their ftrength, and in getting the better of the other ill confequences of the difeafe, than even new-comers. They are likewife more liable to relapfes at various intervals, as two or three weeks, or as many months; but they are not fo violent as in new-comers. They confift ufually of one or two fits of fever, accompanied with ficknefs, retching, and frequently a copious difcharge of bile; from whence fuch patients are commonly faid to be bilious, the bile being fuppofed to be the caufe of the difeafe. The attacks are generally preceded by lofs of appetite, indigeftion, and flatulence in the ftomach and bowels. In the intervals they fometimes enjoy tolerable health, even for years together; more commonly, however, repeated attacks gradually weaken the powers of digeftion in the ftomach, and occafion a remarkable

lofs

lofs of flesh and strength. The complexion grows pale, sallow, and even of a lemon-colour, and the whites of the eyes are clearer than common. In this situation one fit, more violent than the others, shall perhaps put an end at the same time to the patient's life and the disease. Such is the usual manner, in which the disease proves fatal in the natives, and old inhabitants; yet both in them, and in new-comers, it often admits of a speedy solution after two or three fits, and the patient soon recovers completely his ordinary health.

It is worth remarking, that the fever sometimes appears in a very slight way, with languor, lofs of appetite, some degree of head-ach, disturbed sleep, and whitenefs of the tongue, the patient being able all the while to go about his usual employment. In symptoms so moderate the presence of a fever is hardly acknowledged, though the readinefs with which

which they rife into a fevere difeafe, on the leaft irregularity, or any anxiety or diftrefs of mind, leaves no doubt of their nature.

To flight feverifh fymptoms, are fometimes fuperadded, fmall painful tumours in the fkin, called *cat-boils*. They appear to be fmall carbuncles. There is firft a pain felt in the fkin, efpecially on being touched, which is foon followed by a flight fwelling not unlike a common pimple. They are fometimes as large as a nutmeg, and are exceedingly painful, efpecially if fqueezed, or near a joint where there is much motion. They do not fuppurate, but form a kind of core, which is difcharged by one or more holes from the fmall tumour. Any violence applied to them, fuch as attempting to fqueeze the matter out of them, as in a common pimple, produces great fwelling and pain in the furrounding parts. They are confidered as favourable fymptoms,

toms, being supposed to prevent a fever. That however did not appear to be true, for there were many instances of persons being troubled with them for some time, and yet having a fever before they got rid of them. The fever in such cases was not of the most violent kind, though it is not clear that this was owing to the small boils. What might with more certainty be inferred from their presence was, there being a disposition to fever in the constitution for the time. Like the affection of the bowels, they were in one season more prevalent, than in another.

After describing the more usual appearances of the fever, it will not be improper to give some account of those, that were more uncommon.

In some cases the fever begins with fits, like those that happen to children at the eruption of the small pox; and it was only in children that I saw this symptom, though I believe it is not always confined

confined to them. It began in an officer, on the expedition to the Spanish main, with a fainting fit. The jail fever has likewise been observed, to begin with fits in children. This symptom in children, has often given occasion to suspect worms for the cause of the disease, which has led to a dangerous treatment: for what is proper to expel worms will do no good, but on the contrary harm, in the remittent fever.

There is sometimes a great coldness, with a sense of soreness, in a particular part, as the thighs, during the hot fit of the fever, while every other part is parched with heat. Such disagreeable sensations increase the febrile anxiety, and restlessness.

An excruciating pain is sometimes fixed in one part, and follows the fever in its increase and abatement, and after some continuance the part mortifies. I have seen this in the *scrotum*, where I believe

lieve it always proves mortal; and also in the foot, where it was accompanied with a disagreeable sense of coldness, and occasioned the loss of a toe.

In two or three instances the sick complained of a sense of numbness, proceeding sometimes from the head, and sometimes from the stomach, which diffused itself all over the body, and occasioned an extreme alarm while it continued.

Among the symptoms, which more rarely occur, may be mentioned the *tetanus*, and an effusion of water in the ventricles of the brain. The tetanus is of two kinds, one where it is an original disease, another where it is merely a symptom of the fever. It is the latter only of which I am to take notice. The examples of it, which fell under my observation, were few; in one it came after the fever was completely formed, in another it began as soon as the fever. The jaw was locked, and all the joints were rigid, so that the patient placed on his feet was as motionless as a statue. The contractions of the muscles are not equal and uniform at all times, for though they are never relaxed, there are fits of greater and less contraction, and in the former they suffer much pain. The skin is hot, the pulse quick, and the tongue white, when it can be seen; there is also much pain at the pit of the stomach, some degree of stupor, and profuse sweats, particularly about the face.

In one instance of fever, which began in the usual manner, except that the head-ach was greater than common, and appeared to be owing to exposure to the sun, without any covering to the head, after two or three exacerbations a stupor seized the patient; the pupil became dilated, and was almost insensible to the impression of light; he rolled his head about much, and often put his hand to it, with frequent moanings.

moanings. His pulse was about 90 in a minute, and feeble. He remained several days in this state before he died. The body was examined, and there was found about six ounces of limpid *serum* in the ventricles of the brain. The viscera of the thorax, and abdomen, were in a natural state.

Besides the symptoms which more rarely occur during the fever, there are some that follow it, that deserve to be mentioned, though they are not often to be met with. Parotids, or swellings and suppurations of the parotid glands, are sometimes a consequence of the fever; as are also abscesses near the anus, and in other parts of the body. A numbness is at times felt in the arms, for a week or two after the fever; and sometimes flying pains all over the body, like those from rheumatism. There are not wanting examples even of the taste, and smell, being greatly impaired, and remaining so, for several months.

It is not improbable that there may be many more singular, and uncommon symptoms of the fever, than those which have fallen under my observation; yet the sources, from which I derived my experience, must be allowed to have been of the most ample nature, for the space of two years and four months, while I remained with the army in the island of Jamaica, and had the care of the military hospitals there.

It is matter of some consolation, in the history of so grievous a disease, to be able to say with certainty, that it is not infectious. In the military hospitals, the sick admitted with fevers were above three quarters of the whole, and they were often much crowded together, yet there was no reason to believe, that a man with any other complaint, ever caught a fever in the hospital. There was no instance of the yellow fever proving more infectious, than the fever in its more ordinary form, when it was without any change in the colour of the skin. It will not be out of place to remark, that in all the time I was in Jamaica, I saw no instance of the common hospital or jail fever, although many of the military hospitals were very confined; and some of the best of them consisted of a double platform, on which the sick were placed as close together as they could lie. The two diseases are easily distinguished: the disposition to remit, which is constant in the fever of Jamaica, whether with, or without the yellow colour, and which generally shews itself in 36 or 48 hours, with few exceptions, is alone sufficient to discriminate it from the jail or hospital fever. That disease, on the contrary, when once formed, runs its course with great uniformity, and for many days together, there is not the smallest appearance of exacerbation, or remission. The reason, why the

jail

jail fever was not generated in any of the hospitals in Jamaica, was very obvious: every house in the country is constructed so, as to give as free admission to the air as possible, which the great heat of the climate renders necessary. By this means a constant perflation is kept up, and the air that is breathed by the sick changes every moment, and therefore never acquires, by stagnation and confinement, those noxious qualities, which prove the cause of the hospital fever.

As this subject comes to be more investigated, I doubt not but it will be found, that as an hot climate, by rendering ventilation pleasant and agreeable, prevents the jail or hospital fever; so a cold climate, by making it necessary to warm the air artificially, which requires it to be confined to a certain degree, gives rise to the jail or hospital fever; which is not known to proceed from any other cause, except the human species breathing the same

same confined air for some time *, or from such articles of cloathing as retain the poison thus generated. There is no reason to believe, that the generation of the poison is either forwarded, or retarded by the heats or colds of different climates, any farther than as they prove a cause of the confinement, or ventilation of the air, in the apartments of the sick or of others under confinement.

* Vid. Med. Transf. Vol. III. p. 345.

SECT.

SECT. II. *Of the Cure of the Remittent Fever.*

IN treating of the cure of the remittent fever, I shall give an account of the remedies, in the order in which they were administered, when the fever had its most usual appearance; I shall enumerate afterwards, the means that were found most successful in removing, or palliating particular symptoms; and add a few observations on some of the remedies, that have been either strongly recommended, or are in general use.

No disease requires more speedy assistance, for the efficacy of the medicines employed, depends in a great measure on their being given early. The disease gains strength by repeated attacks, and when allowed to have its course, is often fatal. It always greatly impairs the strength, and frequently injures materially the

the conftitution. There is no regular progrefs in the fever, by going through which, the fick are to be reftored to health, and to wait for any *crifis* would be time irrecoverably loft.

If I fee a patient during the firft fit, I direct an ounce of Glauber's falt*, or the fame quantity of the bitter purging falt †, to be diffolved in half a pint of water, to which two drops of the oil of peppermint being added, four table fpoonfuls of the folution are given every half hour, till it operate, or be all taken. As there is generally much ficknefs at ftomach, it is given in fmall dofes, left it fhould excite vomiting. The effential oil covers the tafte of the falt, and renders it lefs offenfive to the ftomach.

It is probably of no great confequence, what kind of purgative medicine is given, provided it operate effectually and without

* Natron vitriolatum, Pharm. Lond. 1788.
† Magnefia vitriolata, Pharm. Lond. 1788.

violence.

violence. Soluble tartar *, Rochel falt †, fena, vitriolated tartar ‡ and rhubarb, or cream of tartar and rhubarb may be ufed, if experience has fhewn that they agree with a particular conftitution. The two purging falts that were firft mentioned, were generally preferred on account of their certain, fpeedy, and eafy operation. Glauber's falt keeps beft in a warm climate; the bitter purging falt attracts moifture and deliquefces, whereby the dofe becomes uncertain, and it is preferved with difficulty.

After a few ftools have been procured, the patient generally finds himfelf much eafier, and a remiffion often enfues. This is to be carefully watched for, and immediate advantage is to be taken of it, for adminiftering the Peruvian bark. The common dofe of this medicine is a drachm,

* Kali tartarifatum, Pharm. Lond. 1788.
† Natron tartarifatum, Pharm. Lond. 1788.
‡ Kali vitriolatum, Pharm. Lond. 1788.

which may be repeated every second hour; and as a general rule in giving it, this is perhaps the beft; but both the quantity and intervals muft often be varied, according to circumftances. Sometimes the ftomach will neither bear fo large a dofe, nor fo frequent a repetition; and therefore, that ficknefs and vomiting may be avoided, the quantity muft be diminifhed to two fcruples, or even half a drachm; and that reduced dofe cannot perhaps be given oftener, than once in three hours. On the contrary, in cafes of great urgency, where the preceding fit has been uncommonly fevere, and there is reafon to fear that the fucceeding one will be ftill more violent, and where a long remiffion cannot be depended upon, the dofe may be increafed to two drachms, which may be given every hour. But few ftomachs will bear fo much, and fometimes the bark cannot be given at all in fubftance. In fuch a cafe recourfe muft be had to a

decoction,

decoction, or an infusion. I prefer the latter, but as the decoction is sooner prepared, I make use of that till the other can be got ready. The infusion is made with two ounces of the best bark, reduced to powder, in twenty-four ounces of cold water; it must be stirred from time to time, and should stand ten or twelve hours, in order to be of a proper strength. Two or three ounces of it are given every two hours, or as often as the stomach will bear it. This preparation taken liberally, has in some instances been more efficacious than the powder itself, for it has prevented a return of fever, when the bark in substance has not afterwards been so successful, in the same person. This I could not easily explain, though I was led to suspect that after one or two violent paroxysms of fever, the stomach was sometimes so weak, that it could not act upon the bark in substance, at least with sufficient power; and that the infusion
found

found a more ready entrance into the circulation. The infusion is lefs offenfive to the ftomach than the decoction, and it is alfo ftronger, if one may judge from the tafte; there is befides no decompofition of the component parts of the bark, which cannot be avoided in the decoction. Such decompofition, it would appear from experiments made by the late Sir John Pringle, much weakens the virtues of the medicine; for, he found that the extract of the bark was not of equal efficacy with the fimple powder, when they were given in the fame quantity.

In fevere attacks of the fever, in which it is abfolutely neceffary to watch for the remiffion, in order to make the beft advantage of it, whenever the pulfe becomes a little flower, and the heat begins to abate, a dofe, or two, of the infufion may be given, and the powder added afterwards as foon, as the ftomach will bear it. This, I found the moft certain way of of moderating, or preventing the next paroxysm.

The vehicle, in which the bark is given, must in many cases be suited to the patient's stomach. It will sometimes sit easy on the stomach when mixed with coffee, with wine and water, or with wine alone, if the remission be considerable; in some cases it answers the same purpose to mix it with milk, or a weak infusion of chamomile flowers. By these expedients, the stomach is reconciled to the medicine, is enabled to receive a larger quantity of it, and to retain it better. If it be not known from experience, what vehicle is the most agreeable, I always make the first trial with the infusion of bark, as being the most efficacious; and if that disagree, recourse is had to the others, till experience teach us which is the best.

It will sometimes happen that the bark purges strongly, and passes through the body

the REMITTENT FEVER.

body almoſt unchanged. This is not an unfavourable ſymptom, and the remedy is eaſy, for three or four drops of the *tinctura thebaica** added to each doſe, ſoon put a ſtop to the purging.

When the method of cure laid down above, is carefully put in practice from the beginning, it will in many caſes prevent a return of the fever; in general, however, a ſufficient quantity of bark cannot be given in the firſt remiſſion, nor is there time for it to produce its effects upon the body, ſo as to prevent a ſecond paroxyſm.

The heat, reſtleſsneſs, anxiety, and indeed all the ſymptoms uſually accompanying the ſecond paroxyſm, are more violent than in the firſt, if nothing has been done in the remiſſion to ſtop the progreſs of the fever; but if the length of the remiſſion, and the ſtate of the ſtomach have admitted of the liberal uſe of

* Tinctura opii, Pharm. Lond. 1788.

the bark, it has a considerable effect upon the ensuing fit. The symptoms run high, but the strength of the patient appears more equal to the struggle; the paroxysm is sharp, but is of shorter duration, and the remission that follows is of the completest kind.

The medicine that I have found most considerably to relieve the symptoms during the paroxysms, and promote a remission, is James's powder. It is given in small doses, seldom exceeding five grains, and is repeated every three or four hours. If the stomach be in an irritable state, the dose is often not larger than half the quantity just mentioned; for, as has been observed before, no symptom of the disease is more troublesome or dangerous than vomiting; in the cure therefore care must be taken to avoid every thing, that might induce or aggravate any tendency that way. The evil that arises from retching and vomiting, is not confined merely to the sufferings of the sick,

the REMITTENT FEVER.

sick, but is most materially felt in preventing the use of such medicines, particularly the bark, as might stop the progress of the disease. The most salutary operation of James's powder is either to excite a sweat, or gently open the body. There is seldom occasion to give James's powder in the first paroxysm, that being occupied by the purgative medicine; but if the fit continue long, as forty-eight hours, and the purge has been given, and produced the full effect, and still there is no remission, James's powder may be given in the manner just mentioned; and by exciting a sweat, or further gently opening the body, it promotes a remission of the fever.

The second remission, as well as the first, is to be employed in administering the bark freely. In this way, above two ounces of the bark may in general be got down, before the period of the fever return, which will in most cases be sufficient

cient either to prevent entirely the next fit, or so far break the force of it, as to render it devoid of danger. In subsequent attacks the same course is to be followed; that is, small doses of James's powder are to be given during the paroxysm, and the bark in the remissions.

If James's powder do not keep the body open, which it seldom fails to do, laxative clysters are of use; for it is to be observed, that one or two stools in the twenty-four hours greatly relieve the sick, and promote the good effects of the bark. This is particularly the case in the fevers subsequent to the rains in September and October, which are of the worst kind. In such, it is frequently advantageous to join four or five grains of rhubarb, to each dose of the bark, in order to procure two or three motions in the day.

I have had occasion to mention, that no symptoms are more dangerous than violent

violent retching and vomiting, and nothing can be more pernicious than the ufe of emetics in fuch circumftances. If there be ficknefs and vomiting in the beginning of the difeafe, chamomile tea, or warm water, are fufficient to cleanfe the ftomach. If the vomiting or retching ftill continue after making ufe of thefe, which they will often do, and harrafs the fick even during a remiffion of the other fymptoms, faline draughts in a ftate of effervefcence, repeated every hour, or oftener, will frequently allay this diftreffing fymptom. The ftomach is alfo relieved by opening the body, which further tends greatly to check the vomiting; but as cathartic medicines would be immediately thrown up, purgative clyfters are the only means that can be employed for that purpofe, and it is fometimes neceffary to repeat them feveral times. In this way the vomiting is often quieted, and the ftomach enabled to retain the bark.

It will sometimes however happen in the worst fevers, that the retchings are not abated by the effervescing draughts, which are themselves thrown up. In such cases I have had recourse to opiates, and generally with success. From fifteen to twenty-five drops of the *tinctura thebaica* * may be added to an effervescing draught, or given in a little Bristol water, and repeated in two or three hours, according to the urgency of the symptoms. In this irritable state of the stomach, Bristol water, either by itself, or mixed with Rhenish wine, or Claret, will often be retained when common water would not. It has been recommended to apply a blister to the epigastric region, when the means above mentioned have failed; but I have never had recourse to it, having always found the vomiting quieted either by the effervescing draught, or the opiate. It must

* Tinct. opii, Pharm. Lond. 1788.

the REMITTENT FEVER. 119

be obvious, that this dangerous symptom will often be induced, and always greatly aggravated, by any method of cure that admits of the use of emetics. The vomiting being overcome, the bark must be given with diligence, yet with caution at first, by beginning with the infusion or decoction, and adding the powder as the stomach will bear it.

During the accession of fever there is commonly more or less of head-ach, which sometimes becomes extremely violent, and greatly distresses the patient. A blister applied between the shoulders, seldom or ever fails either to relieve, or entirely remove this symptom.

In the very low state, that was mentioned sometimes to succeed violent paroxysms, especially in those fevers that were attended with yellowness of the skin, nothing was so useful as cordials; for though the bark was not entirely laid aside, yet the quantity the stomach would bear,

bear, in any form, was so small, that little could be expected from it. Wine and nourishment were the best cordials, and far surpassed any from the shops. Claret and Rhenish wine were most grateful to the sick, and were generally preferred; Madeira was not however refused, if it was desired, and it was the only wine that could be administered in that climate, to the common soldiers. It did not become sour from that kind of treatment, which would have converted any other wine into vinegar. While speaking of this subject, it may be proper to say something of the nourishment, to be given throughout the disease.

During the first attack there is generally a great loathing of food, and of wine; but in the remission this is not the case, and both become requisite in order to support the strength of the patient. Chicken broth, panada, sago, salep, thin gruels, and tea in which bread has

has been foaked, are the kinds of nourifhment beft adapted to the ftate of the ftomach, and to the difeafe. To all of
thefe, except the broth and tea, wine
may be added with fugar and nutmeg, or
any other fpice that is more agreeable.
Wine is feldom to be given by itfelf, but
fhould be mixed with water. In almoft
every cafe, efpecially when the difeafe is
violent, and the patient much reduced,
it is highly grateful and cordial. It is
of the utmoft confequence in giving both
nourifhment and wine, that they be repeated often, and that only a little be
fwallowed at a time; for the ftomach is
eafily overloaded, and provoked to vomit.
After the fever begins to remit, it is
found useful not to give the bark till
fome nourifhment has been taken down,
and of fuch things as are mentioned
above, it is left to the fick to chufe what
is moft agreeable. By this means the
bark fits eafier on the ftomach, and the
fick

sick can better persevere in the use of it. The same purpose is likewise answered by giving some food, or a little wine and water, between every dose of the bark, and the strength of the patient is thereby supported.

When the sick are greatly reduced, after two or more paroxysms of fever, wine and nourishment become more essential than medicine; for in such circumstances the bark itself does little or no good, till the powers of life are in some degree recruited. If it be not entirely laid aside therefore, it should only be given in a cold infusion, to the quantity of three or four spoonfuls, and repeated once in two or three hours; the powder is to be added gradually as the sick can bear it, and in such manner as not to oppress or load the stomach, which would impede the use of wine and nourishment. It is of the last importance, to give the sick in this way,

proper

proper nourishment from time to time; for, though they have no call for it, if it be omitted for even a short time, they grow gradually weaker and weaker, the pulse often indicating no return of fever, and expire, as if the whole powers of life were exhausted by the preceding paroxysm.

It may be asked, in what quantity should wine be given? It is difficult to give a precise answer to this; the quantity must bear a proportion to it's effects, and I have generally been guided by the following circumstances. If it be not grateful to the sick, but on the contrary disagreeable, it will seldom do good; nor is it attended with better effects, if it increase the heat, restlessness, or delirium. When it agreed well with the sick, I have in general found the quantity, that had the best effects, much less than what is often recommended. I have rarely given above a pint in the twenty-four hours, and from watching it's effects, was well assured, that going beyond that quantity would

would have done no good, but on the contrary, harm. I do not speak of the jail fever, in which wine has been recommended, and given in very large quantities; although my experience even in that disease, has not furnished me with cases, where the quantity could be made with safety, much to exceed that mentioned above. It happens most unfortunately in physic, that we can hardly correct one error without rushing into another; not content with substituting wine and cordials in the room of evacuations, we must produce intoxication, without considering that in all cases, where the human body is greatly reduced or exhausted, the strength and quantity even of cordials must bear a direct proportion, to the remaining strength of the sick.

If the thirst be great, and not quenched by the thin liquors mentioned above, the sick are allowed to drink water, or toast and water. When the stomach is extremely

tremely irritable and difposed to vomit, Briftol water is often more grateful than any other liquor, and frequently ftays upon the ftomach, when nothing elfe will. Acid, or acefcent liquors, prepared from the fruits of the country have been extravagantly recommended, as highly grateful to the fick, and falutary in the difeafe; but fuch encomiums appear to be the refult rather of hypothefis, than experience. The fick have in general no craving for them, and when given they frequently produce uneafinefs at ftomach. There is often indeed a difpofition to fournefs in the ftomach, as appears from the green colour, and four fmell, of what is thrown up, and this fymptom is aggravated by acefcent liquors.

It fometimes happens during the paroxyfm of the fever, that there is a confiderable degree of *ftupor* or *coma*, which, in fome cafes, rifes to almoft a total infenfibility.

sibility. This being a symptom of the fever, whatever is useful in procuring a remission, helps to remove it. For this particular purpose, I have not learned any thing more effectual than James's powder, which may be given more liberally in such cases, as in general the stomach is not in an irritable state. It may be given in the dose of five grains, and repeated every second, or third hour, till the fever remit, or the medicine have some sensible operation. A stupor or coma is a mark of a severe disease, and strongly indicates the necessity of making the best use of the ensuing remission, by giving the bark in the most effectual manner, in order to check or moderate the next paroxysm, which otherwise might prove fatal.

In treating the sick, I have supposed the method of cure, to be put in practice from the beginning of the disease; but this cannot always be the case, as, for various and obvious reasons, a first or even a second

the REMITTENT FEVER.

a second paroxysm may have passed, before any thing is done towards the cure. In this situation, if there be a remission, and the preceding fit has been violent, and there is reason to suspect that the subsequent one will be more so, it is not advisable to lose three, or four hours, in giving an opening medicine, which must therefore be omitted, and the bark administered directly. In order, however, to prevent any sense of fulness, either in the stomach or bowels, which might arise from that medicine, and likewise to promote the operation of it upon the constitution, some opening medicine is joined to it, so as to procure three or four stools in the twenty-four hours. With this view four, or five grains of rhubarb, may be added to each dose of the bark.

If a delirium, with a considerable degree of wildness and agitation, which sometimes prevail during the paroxysm, continue after the usual evacuations, an opiate

opiate given in a moderate dose, and repeated after two or three hours, will in some cases have a good effect in quieting it, and thereby promote a remission of the fever.

A large quantity of wind is sometimes generated in the bowels, producing considerable distension and pain. Clysters, and gentle laxatives, by promoting the expulsion of it, give relief. A drop of oil of peppermint upon a bit of sugar, or two or three spoonfuls of the *Julepum e Camphora* *, procure temporary ease. Though it be a desirable thing to remove this symptom, yet it is not of consequence enough to interrupt the use of the bark, and it will generally be sufficient to add as much rhubarb to that medicine, as will keep the body open.

In the history of the symptoms it was mentioned, that there was sometimes a

---

* Mistura camphorata, Pharm. Lond. 1788.

soreness

soreness of the flesh, as if beat or bruised. In one case, this was particularly felt in the thighs, which were besides cold, even during the height of the fever, though the legs and feet were hot. The pain and uneasiness were considerable, and occasioned great restlessness and anxiety in the patient. A *semicupium* was used, but the patient's strength would not permit a continuance of it, so as to procure relief. Flannels wrung from boiling water were wrapt so hot round the thighs, that they could not be born by any other part of the body, yet they proved pleasant and gave great ease. A fomentation of this kind was continued for a considerable time, till the fever began to remit, which it seemed much to promote by the ease it procured.

It sometimes happens that there is a pain confined to one spot, with a sense of coldness in the part; and after one or more fits of fever the part mortifies, becoming

becoming livid and dead. Inſtances of this occured in the *ſcrotum* and foot, as has been mentioned. Of thoſe affected in the former, I knew of none that recovered; in a caſe of the latter, warm fomentations, and bottles filled with hot water applied to the part affected, gave conſiderable relief. Opiates did no good. When the part became livid and inſenſible, it was ſcarified, in order to diſcharge a thin ichorous matter, which procured ſome eaſe. The fever was checked by the uſe of bark, and the patient recovered, with the loſs of one toe; but he was ſubject to relapſes for a long time, and did not regain his ſtrength for ſeveral months.

When a ſeaſon proves unhealthy, more particularly at the moſt ſickly time of the year, relapſes are very frequent. They are ſometimes ſlight, ſometimes ſevere, but never devoid of danger; for repeated attacks undermine the conſtitution, and end

end in dropfies, or indurations of the liver or fpleen; or perhaps one fit, more fevere than ufual, puts an end to the life of the patient. In fuch cafes the treatment, during the fever, is the fame as is laid down above; that is, an opening medicine in the beginning, James's powder as occafion may require to haften a remiffion, and afterwards the bark : for it is to be obferved, that thofe relapfes confift of two or more feverifh fits, and remiffions between. When the conftitution becomes liable to relapfes, which fometimes take place with a degree of regularity every two, three, or four weeks, it is of great advantage to procure a change of air, or what is ftill better, repeated changes of it by travelling. Eafy journies in the cooler and mountainous part of the country, continued for fome time, are very efficacious in reftoring ftrength and vigour to the conftitution;

and in enabling it to refift future returns of the diforder.

The air of Port Royal, which ftands upon a bank of fand, that is nearly furrounded by the fea, is pure and healthy, and is frequently of great benefit to invalids, from the neighbouring towns of Kingfton and Spanifh Town; though in the temperature of the air there be little difference between the three places. Port Royal would be ftill more healthy, were due attention given to remove dirt and filth from the ftreets.

Such however is the deep root that the fever fometimes takes, that the relief procured by a change of air is of fhort duration, and repeated attacks ftill threaten to prove fatal. Under fuch circumftances a fea voyage is highly beneficial, and will often accomplifh what a change of air alone could not; efpecially if the time of being at fea can be prolonged to ten or twelve weeks. It was
imagined

the REMITTENT FEVER. 133

imagined at one time, that this might have been turned to the advantage of the common foldiers, by fending the convalefcents to make a cruize on board the fhips of war; and fome men, belonging to the 1ft battalion of the 60th regiment, were accordingly fent to fea. But being unable to lay in fea ftock, and not knowing how to take care of themfelves on board of fhip, they all returned with the fcurvy, though free from fever; upon which the plan was laid afide.

The air at fea, in the Weft Indies, is free from all the pernicious qualities of the air on fhore, and there is no climate where feamen enjoy better health, provided they remain conftantly on board of fhip, and attention be paid to keep the fhip clean, and to fupply the men from time to time with vegetables or fruits, to prevent the fcurvy. The finenefs of the weather makes it feldom neceffary to fhut the port-holes, and therefore they do not suffer from foul and confined air; and almost all the islands afford supplies of fruits, greens, and esculent roots. The ships of war, on the Jamaica station, often enjoy better health than in the English Channel. This being the case, it may be asked how it happens that we lose so many of our seamen in the West Indies? It is owing to the following causes, as far as I could observe, on the Jamaica station, to which my remarks particularly refer, though, I doubt not, they will equally apply to the other islands.

Sailors when sent on shore, either for the purpose of taking in water, or on any other duty, are exposed to the causes that produce the fevers of the country; and in general they give additional efficacy to them, by their own irregularities. It would further seem, that coming from a pure air into one that is noxious, they are nearly in the same situation as new-comers,

comers, who are sooner affected, and suffer more from fevers than others, as was mentioned before. In taking in water, at the watering-place for the navy, in the harbour of Kingston, it has frequently happened, that every man employed on that service has been seized with a fever, in the course of a few days; and although this be not always the case, it is very rare that the larger proportion do not suffer. Again, the men of war supply the deficiency of their complement by pressing the sailors from the merchant ships; to avoid which, many of the men leave their ships as soon as they make the land, and lurk in the country or towns, till an opportunity offer of getting on board a trading ship, or till they fall into the hands of a press-gang. Those men, as well as the sailors employed in the pressing duty, are all exposed to the usual causes of sickness, and after going on board the king's ships, many of them are

are seized with fevers. This has been particularly remarked, in those ships that have been manned entirely in Jamaica; which happened, when ships taken from the enemy were bought into the service of government; and upon some occasions of this kind, the mortality has not been less among the officers than the men, owing, apparently, to the former having taken an active part in the pressing service. I am not ignorant that it has been supposed, that the foul state of the ships taken from the enemy, has produced contagious fevers, to which the mortality alluded to has been imputed. But it is worthy of remark, that there was no contagious fever among the enemies' men, while on board the same ships; and that though they were dirty, there was no confined air, and it is the latter only that is known to produce contagious fevers. But what appears to be of more force than either of those arguments is, that

that many of those who died had the yellow fever, which is sufficiently characteristic of the distemper of the country, and is an appearance rarely to be met with in contagious fevers.

Besides the pressing and the watering services, there are many smaller matters that render it necessary to send boats ashore, and without particular care the men will straggle into the country, or about the towns, which is rarely done with impunity, especially at the unhealthy season of the year. Ships may likewise become unhealthy, though none of their men go on shore, if stationed near to marshy ground, and to leeward of it. To those causes, which introduce fevers into the fleet, may be added another source of the mortality, which prevails among our sailors in the West Indies, that the surgeons of the navy are not supplied with the most essential medicine for their cure, at least in proper quantity;
I mean

I mean the Peruvian bark: nor can they afford to purchafe it in that part of the world*.

Having thus ftated fhortly, the principal caufes of mortality, in the fleet in the Weft Indies, it will not be deemed digreffing too far, to mention in a few words the remedies that may be ufed to counteract them.

I. Sailors fhould not be allowed to go on fhore, when it can poffibly be avoided.

II. Negroes fhould be employed for the watering fervice.

III. The furgeons fhould have an allowance of bark from government, while upon that ftation.

In order the better to reconcile the failors to remain on board of fhip, while in harbour, market boats under proper regulations fhould not only be allowed, but encouraged to come to the fhip, that they may have an opportunity of laying

* It fometimes fells for two guineas a pound.

out their prize-money, in whatever articles they pleafe, that are not pernicious to them.

The purchafe of Negroes for the watering fervice would be confiderable, but nothing when compared to the lofs fuftained by the death of fo many feamen, rating them merely at the expence they coft government, and laying afide fuch confiderations as are derived from humanity. The life of a failor in the Weft Indies cannot be rated at lefs than fifty pounds; and even at that computation, which is much too low, the number loft in watering a few line of battle fhips, far exceeds the expence of purchafing negroes. But a fufficient number might be provided with no additional expence, if every fhip were to have a certain proportion of negroes, according to their complement, as one in twenty or twenty-five. They might be hired of their mafters, or entered if free, and turned over by the
fhips

ships leaving the station, to those that arrived there. A similar practice is found very useful in the army. All the negroes, on board the ship in the harbour, might when needful be employed in filling water; nor would they, like Europeans, suffer from fevers; for, though not entirely exempted from that disease, they are but slightly affected by it.

The expence of supplying the navy surgeons with bark, is too inconsiderable to be any just bar to a plan, which has for its object, a matter of so much consequence, as that of saving the lives of our seamen.

To return to our subject, a voyage to sea often entirely restores the health, and seldom or ever fails to procure a considerable temporary amendment. Should however the fever still return in a formidable way, there is but one thing remaining to be done, which is, to go to a colder climate, either in Europe or North America.

America. The health is generally much improved during the voyage, and in a cooler and more healthy climate, is often completely re-eſtabliſhed in a few months. But this is not always the caſe, for the conſtitution is ſometimes ſo materially injured, as not to admit of a ſpeedy reſtoration. The ſick remain ſubject to returns of fever, at various intervals, for the ſpace of ſix, twelve, or even eighteen months after their arrival in Europe. The attacks, it is true, are neither ſo violent, nor ſo frequent as they would have been in the Weſt Indies, but ſtill they are conſiderable enough to prevent the recovery of ſtrength, and to keep the ſick in a ſtate of great languor and dejection. During the feveriſh fits the ſtomach and bowels are often much difordered, and if vomiting be excited, more or leſs of bile is brought up, and from this circumſtance ſuch perſons are ſaid to be bilious. The ſalutary influence of a cold climate will, in moſt caſes, gradually reſtore health ;

the

the good effects of it are however promoted by gentle exercife, in the open air when the weather is fine, as riding on horfeback; by opening medicines of an eafy operation, during the attacks of fever; by the occafional ufe of bitters, bark, and chalybeate medicines to ftrengthen the ftomach, and conftitution; and by fea-bathing during the warmer months.

To return to the treatment of the fever in Jamaica, it was mentioned that the bowels were at times affected with dyfenteric fymptoms: if they were flight, they fometimes yielded to the purgative given in the beginning; but when they did not, fomething of an opening nature, as a few grains of rhubarb, was added to the bark. If the affection of the bowels did not give way to this, and the dyfentery might be faid to conftitute the principal difeafe, the method of cure was the fame as will be mentioned, in treating of that difeafe.

When there was a combination of cat-boils with fever, the former required no particular treatment; care however was to be taken that no violence was offered to them; for if an attempt was made to squeeze them, or if they were near a joint that was necessarily much in motion, as the elbow-joint, they became excessively painful, inflamed all round, and formed a real carbuncle.

Of the tetanus, as a symptom of fever, I have little to observe. The methods of cure hitherto recommended in every species of this disease, are at least uncertain, if not altogether inefficacious. A new remedy answered well in one case, and although little can be inferred therefrom, it may deserve to be noticed in a complaint, where our knowledge is so limited. It consisted of an electuary made of the flower of mustard * and common

---

* I was led to make trial of this in consequence of a conversation with the late Dr. H. Saunders, who said he had heard it had done good in tetanus.

syrup,

syrup, of which one or two tea spoonfuls were given every two hours, or even every hour if the throat and stomach would bear it. In two days the symptoms yielded, the patient could open his jaw, and the rigidity of his limbs and body went off; the medicine was therefore laid aside. But in less than two days the symptoms recurred, the electuary was given as before, and again the disease seemed to yield to it. Whether this was to be ascribed to the medicine, or was merely fortuitous, must be determined by future trials. Hippocrates orders black hellebore and pepper in this disease *.

In the case of hydrocephalus, that was a consequence of the fever, blisters to the forehead, temples, and back were ineffectually applied; and it was intended to have given *calomel* in small doses, as the most probable means of promoting an

* De Morbis, lib. iii.

absorption

absorption of the water, but the patient died before a trial of it could be made.

The fever has many intermediate degrees of violence, between the severe attack that puts an end to life in one or two days, and a form so slight, that the presence of a fever is hardly suspected. There is lassitude, a want of the usual appetite for food, disturbed sleep, and, what is chiefly characteristic of the fever, a white tongue. Such symptoms will continue for several days, without giving any alarm, though they are always ready to be converted into a severe illness, when aided by an additional cause. A dose of physick will often remove them all, and a gentle emetic will frequently have the same effect; but the former was commonly preferred, as being fully more effectual, and easier in its operation. James's powder, given in the quantity of eight or ten grains at bed-time, and repeated for two or three nights, will often

often restore the health, without producing any sensible operation. One particular advantage derived from it, is to take off the heat and restlessness, which are often extremely troublesome in the night. Travelling by easy journeys, or making short excursions from the usual place of residence, are highly beneficial, and will often completely re-establish the health.

Before I conclude, it may be allowed to observe, that the practice had two leading objects in view; to procure a remission; and to prevent a return of the fever. The first was obtained chiefly by opening medicines, and James's powder; the second was accomplished by the bark in different forms. The advantages of this practice over that, in which more time is spent in cleansing the *primæ viæ*, as it is expreſt, and where the first remission is usually sacrificed to that purpose, are, that the fever is sooner checked, the constitution of the patient suffers less,

the

the recovery of strength is quicker and more complete, and relapses happen less frequently. The longer the fever continues, the more mischief is done; nor is there the smallest appearance of its having a regular progress towards a crisis, to wait for which would be time irretrievably lost. The means of cure are few and simple; the greatest difficulty is in watching the proper times of using them, and in administering them with diligence and assiduity. I found them so seldom disappoint me, that there were few besides of the long list of medicines, usually recommended in fevers, to which I had recourse. As the practice however was not reduced all at once to so much simplicity, but at first trials were made of several of the remedies in common use, it may not be improper to mention shortly the results of them.

 Blood-letting well deserves to be considered in the first place. In such cases as seemed most to require it, for example, where the patient was young, strong, of a full habit, and lately arrived from Europe; where the pulse was quick and full, the face flushed with great heat and head-ach, and all these at the beginning of the fever, bleeding did no good. It neither diminished the symptoms for the time, nor procured a speedier remission. I cannot say, however, that it did that mischief that has been imputed to it by some; for, provided it were in a moderate quantity, it could hardly be said to produce any ill consequences. But if it were copious, or repeated a second time, it was always hurtful, and rendered the recovery of the patient extremely slow, if not attended with worse consequences. This effect it had in the inflammations of the lungs that sometimes happened, in which it was necessary to bleed freely. It will not be considered as a recommendation of bleeding to say, that there were some fome cafes in which it did little or no harm, if ufed moderately; yet fuch is the conclufion, to which the obfervations I had an opportunity of making lead me. The general ufe of copious bleedings in fevers, in which there is no local inflammation, would indeed appear to have been introduced into practice upon hypothetical principles. A fever was fuppofed to depend upon a fermentation in the blood and humours, whereby great commotions were excited, like to what happens in other fermenting liquors, and by drawing off part of the blood, there was more room for the remainder to go through the procefs of fermentation, and defpumation. Sydenham * gave fome fanction to thefe ill-founded opinions, and they were afterwards carried to greater lengths, and wrought into a fyftem by the genius of Boerhaave †, in

* Sydenham, Febr. Contin. an. 1661, 62, 63, 64.
† Boerhaave Aphorifm. 615.

whose school it was an axiom, almost without exception, to bleed in the beginning of fevers.

Vomits are much used in fevers in the present practice, but I did not find them of advantage in the remittent Fever of Jamaica; on the contrary, when that disease is violent, the worst symptom is a retching or vomiting, which is greatly aggravated by emetics; and under such circumstances they are inadmissible. But when the stomach is not in an irritable state, and there is little or no disposition to vomiting, it is easily excited by an emetic, and often allayed with difficulty. In all cases a vomit ruffled and fatigued the patient more than a purge, without procuring equal relief; and if a vomit were given during the paroxysm of the fever, it was generally deemed necessary afterwards to give a purgative, before the bark could be administered; by which a whole remission was often lost. The notion

notion entertained by some, that bile is the cause of the fever, led to a frequent use of vomits, and sometimes with the most pernicious effects; for the stomach was rendered so irritable thereby, that wine, nourishment, or even a glass of water could not be retained, but were thrown up almost as soon as swallowed. Emetics given in small doses, and repeated at short intervals, so as to excite and keep up for some time a nausea or sickness at stomach, were not less pernicious than when employed for the purpose of evacuating the bile. In either case the stomach was rendered incapable of receiving the bark, the only medicine we are yet acquainted with, that possesses power to stop the progress of the fever.

I did not find, that I could by any means contrive to give the emetic tartar so, as to produce the same effects as James's powder; the peculiar advantage of which is, that it does not so readily affect the stomach as emetic tartar, but operates chiefly by purging, or sweating. These effects probably depend upon its being a calx, and not a saline preparation, of antimony. Saline preparations affect the stomach directly, whereas a calx acts slowly, and passes into the bowels before it produces its full operation. James's powder appears, however, to be superior to any preparation of the *antimonium calcinatum*, that we are yet acquainted with, which is probably owing to the process by which it is made, being of that kind that determines exactly the degree of calcination, upon which the virtues of antimonials are known chiefly to depend.

The red Peruvian bark was not found more effectual than the common kind; on the contrary, there were considerable objections to the use of it in the cure of the remittent fever. It frequently affected the stomach and bowels, producing sickness, ficknefs, and fometimes vomiting, with flatulence, griping, and purging. Thofe effects were often troublefome, and retarded the cure; the common bark was therefore, after making comparative trials, preferred to the red bark. The prejudices, that formerly exifted againft the Peruvian bark, are no longer in being. They were founded in idle fpeculations, and originated with the learned, from whom they defcended to the great body of the people; but even with the vulgar they are now extinct. Any attempt to prove, that the obftructions of the *vifcera* are the effects of the difeafe, and not of the medicine, would at this time be deemed impertinent. The greateft and indeed the only evil arifing from the bark, that has fallen under my obfervation, has been to excite ficknefs, naufea, and vomiting, when it has difagreed with the ftomach. Thofe effects it generally produces, if it be given during the paroxyfm of the fever.

ver. An anxiety to administer early this great specific, sometimes led to a practice of that kind, but nothing was gained by it, as it was almost always rejected by the stomach. Nay, there was some danger of raising a disgust in the patient to the medicine, which might continue during the remission.

Blisters were often applied by some in the cure of the fever. It will be obvious, that there must be a degree of uncertainty, in appreciating the effects of a remedy, which does not complete its operation in less than twelve or fifteen hours, in a disease that consists of remissions and exacerbations, following each other at no fixed or regular periods. Under such circumstances, remissions must often occur during the operation of the blisters, but there was no reason to think that they were promoted by them; and the blisters certainly had no effect in preventing future attacks of fever. In cases of great stupor

the REMITTENT FEVER. 155

ftupor and infenfibility, where it might have been expected they would have been moft ufeful, they did no good. When the fever was violent, and the paroxyfms long, it frequently happened that the blifters rofe well, and produced their full effect, yet the fever went on, as if no fuch application had been made. Finding that they neither fhortened the fit, nor prevented future returns; that the difcharge from them was often fo confiderable, from the diffolved ftate of the blood, as greatly to weaken the fick; that they frequently produced ulcers that were healed with much difficulty, and fometimes mortifications that proved fatal; I laid afide the ufe of them entirely, unlefs the fick were diftreffed with a bad headach, for which fymptom they were in fome fort a fpecific. The fame objections were found to hold good againft fynapifms.

The clafs of alexipharmic and cordial
medicines,

medicines, I made little or no use of, having found wine to be not only more grateful to the sick, but also much more effectual in answering all the purposes, for which such medicines are given.

Sect. III. *Of the Nature and Causes of the Remittent Fever.*

I have purposely avoided conjectural, or speculative reasoning on this disease, and have confined myself to a simple narrative of symptoms, appearances, and effects of medicine, as learned from observation and experience. Theoretical disquisitions, into the nature and causes of diseases, have often done much mischief, and seldom any good. Our knowledge of the animal economy is hitherto so limited, that it enables us to make little or no progress in such undertakings; and analogies

analogies from chemiftry, mechanics, and other fciences, however well imagined, or fpecioufly decorated, have been found unequal to the explanation of the *phænomena* of living bodies. It may be a queftion, whether all fuch inveftigations fhould not be excluded from the ftudy of phyfic; and there are many that would not hefitate to anfwer in the affirmative. But there is confiderable difficulty in this; the mind cannot make obfervations without comparing them, without tracing their refemblances, and marking their relations; and unlefs reftrained by the laws of true philofophy, it haftens to conclufions that muft be erroneous, becaufe derived from inadequate *data*. Hence it has happened from the earlieft annals of Phyfic, that there have been various opinions, generally derived from the philofophy of the times, which have been adopted as principles, from which the nature and caufes of difeafes

might

might be explained. It is my intention, rather to examine the opinions of this kind, that are entertained respecting the remittent fever, than to advance any notions of my own. If it be considered, that the received idea, of the cause of a disease, has generally great influence in directing the practice, the present inquiry will hardly be thought labour misemployed.

That the bile is the cause of the remittent fever, is an opinion more commonly received than any other; it is of the highest antiquity. In a disease that usually begins with sickness and vomiting, the discharge of a fluid possessing such peculiar properties, both as to taste and colour as the bile, could not fail to make a strong impression on the first observers. It was natural for them to conclude that, that fluid, which they had seen nothing of while the body continued in an healthy state, was the cause of the

the difeafe; and the relief the fick are fenfible of, from the fweating that ufually follows the retching and vomiting, and the confequent difcharge of bile, would confirm them in this opinion. It could not be long, however, before they would learn that the bile was a natural fecretion, which was conftantly going on in an healthy ftate, and therefore that the fever could not be imputed fimply to the prefence of bile, for then nobody would be without a fever. It was fuppofed, that the bile was in fault either in quantity, or in particular acquired qualities. It was either acrimonious, putrid, or in too large a quantity; or perhaps faulty in all thofe refpects. Such are the opinions delivered by the oldeft medical writers, and they are received by many of the prefent day with little variation, and confidered as applying particularly to the remittent fever.

That the bile in a natural ftate is perfectly

fectly harmless, at least as far as relates to fevers, we have daily proofs, in its being most intimately diffused all over the body in jaundice, without exciting any febrile disorder. The proofs of this fluid being in a putrid, or acrimonious state, are taken from the changes it undergoes in colour and consistence. The natural colour of it is yellow, but it is often vomited green, and sometimes of a dark brown colour, or almost black, and of a ropy consistence. The quantity has generally been supposed to exceed what is natural; yet I apprehend it is not an easy matter to ascertain, how much bile is secreted in an healthy person, and unless that could be done, it is difficult to say, at what point the quantity discharged, exceeds that of the healthy secretion.

The green colour of the bile is known to depend upon an acid in the stomach; for experiments have taught us, that the most

most healthy bile would acquire a green colour, if mixed with an acid liquor. That an acid is often generated in the stomach we have daily proofs, both in the four taste of what is brought up from the stomach, and in the teeth being set on edge by it. I have seen an instance of fever, in which it was necessary to give from half an ounce to six drachms of the powder of oyster-shells, to destroy the acid that was generated in the course of the day, which otherwise occasioned great pain and retchings. The green colour therefore is not to be imputed to any acrimony, or other bad quality in the bile, but to a disease in the stomach.

The dark brown colour of the bile, and ropy consistence, are nothing more than natural changes, produced by its stagnating for some time in the gall-bladder and biliary ducts. The thinner parts of the bile are absorbed, and what remains becomes both of a deeper colour, and thicker consistence, confiftence, as happens in other fecretions.

The bile is not a fluid that has a ftrong tendency to putrefaction, but the contrary; and there are no facts to prove that it is ever thrown up from the ftomach in a putrid ftate; it is not therefore confiftent with the rules of juft reafoning, to fuppofe fuch a ftate for the purpofe of explaining the *phænomena*.

The great quantity of bile, that is often difcharged, is to be attributed to the retching and vomiting. In fea-ficknefs the quantity of bile that is thrown up, is often as confiderable as in the remittent fever, yet it cannot be fuppofed to be the caufe of fea-ficknefs or vomiting, but, on the contrary, is the effect of them; and, though difcharged moft profufely, is never accompanied with any fever. A vomit, that operates ftrongly, never fails to bring up a large quantity of bile, which does not appear till after repeated

peated ftrainings and retchings: the ufual contents of the ftomach are firft difcharged, and after a time the bile. The progrefs is the fame in the remittent fever, the contents of the ftomach are firft thrown up, and if the vomiting continue, the bile afterwards makes its appearance. So far, therefore, is it from being the caufe of the ficknefs and vomiting, that it does not even find its way into the ftomach, till the ftraining has continued fome time. The large quantity thrown up may depend on two caufes; the violent vomiting, which in all cafes excites a moft copious flow of bile; and the operation of digeftion being at a ftand, the flow of the bile into the duodenum is not promoted; for the diftenfion of the ftomach by the food occafions a compreffion of the gall-bladder, which not taking place, the bile is collected in a large quantity, and when vomiting comes to be excited, is of courfe more copiously discharged. It is in this way that Morgagni * explains, how the gall-bladder is found distended with bile after death; but I am inclined to think that there are other circumstances, that should be taken into the account. Glands, and excretory ducts have their peculiar *stimuli,* which throw them into action, and produce a copious flow of their secreted liquors. Thus, the saliva flows as soon as any thing sapid or grateful is taken into the mouth; and tears run from the eyes when certain pungent effluvia fill the nostrils, such being sufficient to excite the action of the lachrymal glands. There is reason to think that the same principle holds in the more internal glands, whose operations we cannot so well observe; and that the food taken into the stomach excites the secretion of the gastric juices, and after passing through

---

* Morgagni de Sedibus & Causis Morb. Ep. 68. § 3.

the pylorus proves a ſtimulus equally powerful, in promoting the flow of the pancreatic juice and bile into the duodenum, there to be mixed and blended together, for purpoſes in the animal œconomy, which we do not yet underſtand. It is probable therefore, that this natural action contributes more to the evacuation of the gall-bladder, than any mechanical preſſure of the ſtomach; and when digeſtion is at a ſtand, the bile of courſe will accumulate, till it be diſcharged by vomiting or purging. The collection and ſtagnation of the bile produce the deep colour and ropy conſiſtence, which it ſometimes acquires. It deſerves to be remarked, that in the ſtage of the fever which is moſt commonly imputed to bile, the firſt marks of the diſeaſe are loſs of appetite and ſlight ſickneſs at ſtomach *, which are often preſent for a

* Vide p. 94.

whole day before the attack of fever, and during that time the bile is collecting, and accumulates in the ducts and gall-bladder.

Thus, the quantity of the bile, as well as its suppofed bad qualities, depending upon caufes that have no neceffary connection with the remittent fever, and occurring wherever thofe caufes are to be met with, even where there is no fever, it is not allowable to impute to bile, or any change it is yet known to undergo, the production of remittent fevers. There are not wanting other proofs to fhew, that the difcharge of bile is merely an accidental fymptom; for cafes frequently occur where no bile is thrown up at all, and yet the fever is as regularly formed, and as violent, as when that fluid is difcharged in large quantities. Indeed the difcharge of bile is often intirely owing to the ufe of emetics, and is always greatly increafed by them. It would be of little

little moment to inveſtigate this ſubject, did it not involve opinions productive of the worſt conſequences, in the treatment of the diſeaſe. If bile, whether putrid, acrid, or ſuperabundant, be the cauſe of fever, can any thing be ſo proper as to promote the diſcharge and evacuation of it by vomits? Emetics, therefore, upon this ground are given, and repeated; and as bile is diſcharged every time, an argument is thence deduced for their future repetitions; without reflecting that while life remains, a ſtrong vomit will always bring up bile, in the ſame manner that any irritation upon the eye would produce a flow of tears. But in the remittent fever of Jamaica there is not room for many repetitions of vomiting, except in ſlight caſes indeed; for the irritability of the ſtomach peculiar to the diſeaſe, if increaſed by an emetic, renders it impoſſible for a time, to adminiſter any medicine to check the progreſs of the fever, and a second or third attack under such circumstances will generally prove fatal.

While it has been generally agreed to consider the bile as the cause of the remittent fever, a symptom of the disease so remarkable as to give rise to a new name, I mean the yellowness of the skin, in consequence of which it is called the *yellow fever*, has been derived from another source, and not imputed to the bile; though that be the only cause we are hitherto acquainted with, which produces a yellowness of the skin. The colour of the skin, in the yellow fever, has been supposed to arise from a putrid and dissolved state of the blood.

In speaking of the symptoms of the disease, it was observed, that the yellowness first appeared in the eyes, then upon the neck and shoulders, and at last all over the body, holding exactly the same progress as in the jaundice. At the same time that
the

the skin becomes yellow, the urine is voided of a deep colour, and tinges a bit of linen rag yellow, as in the jaundice. When the sick recover from the fever, the colour gradually disappears as in that disease. The progress of the symptoms, as far as respects the yellow colour, being exactly similar in the remittent fever and the jaundice, it is consistent with reason to believe, that the colour proceeds from the same cause in both, that is, from the bile being absorbed, and carried by the lymphatic vessels into the general mass of circulating fluids. In jaundice the bile is absorbed when the ducts, that should convey it into the duodenum, are obstructed. The most common cause of obstruction is undoubtedly biliary *calculi* or concretions, and sometimes scirrhous tumours compressing the ducts. It is not so obvious, what the cause of obstruction is in the remittent fever; but before hazarding any conjecture upon that head, it it may not be improper to confider, what foundation there is for the opinion, that the yellow colour depends upon a putrid or diffolved ftate of the blood.

Without examining whether the term *putrid* can be applied with propriety to the blood, while in the living body, the prefent queftion may be confined to this point; how far the yellow colour can be produced by any change of the blood, whether induced by putrefaction, or a diffolution of its fubftance. A putrid and diffolved ftate of the blood, as it is commonly expreffed, occurs chiefly in the advanced ftages of fea-fcurvy, in certain fevers, and in fome morbid and undefcribed conditions of the body. In all thofe the blood is known to be in a diffolved ftate, by oozing through the veffels, and fometimes through the pores of the fkin, and producing fpots of various kinds upon the fkin. There is perhaps no difeafe, in which the blood is in a

more

more diffolved ftate, than in the fea-fcurvy; yet it never produces a yellow colour of the fkin in that difeafe, The difcolouring is not uniform, but in fpots or wheals, which are at firft red or a purplifh black, or of fome intermediate fhade, the colour being more or lefs deep according to the quantity of blood that is effufed. The fame thing is obfervable in the diffolved ftate of the blood, that happens in fevers; and in neither is the colour of the eye affected. When the fpots begin to difappear they leave indeed a yellow tinge in the fkin, like to what happens after a bruife; but this yellownefs is confined to the fpots, has a marbled appearance, and is not generally diffufed over the fkin. The diffolved, or as it is called, putrid ftate of the blood, being incapable of producing the yellow colour in the eyes and fkin, and the abforption of the bile being the only caufe we are hitherto acquainted with that can produce thofe effects,

fects, there is good ground to conclude, that it is the cause of the yellowness, and that the yellow fever is in no other respects to be distinguished from the remittent fever, than in having a jaundice superadded.

Next to the opinion that the fever proceeds from bile, none is more prevalent than that it is of a putrid nature; and that the whole mass of humours are running violently into putrefaction. If it be asked what is meant by the term *putrefaction*, it will doubtless be answered, that species of fermentation or change, which dead animal matter in a certain degree of heat and moisture, joined to an admission of air, spontaneously undergoes. That such is the acceptation of the term cannot be doubted, when it is observed that in reasoning on this subject, whatever is found to check putrefaction out of the body, is supposed to have the same effect taken internally.

ternally, and is therefore recommended in difeafes believed to be putrid; and whatever promotes putrefaction out of the body, is fuppofed to be noxious, and is therefore avoided. Putrefaction diffolves bodies, and the diffolution is accompanied with an offenfive fmell. In the fever, the blood is fometimes in a diffolved ftate, and there often proceeds from the body of the fick a peculiar fmell, extremely difagreeable: fo far there is a refemblance, but it goes no farther. In the dead body the firft figns of putrefaction are an offenfive fmell, and change of colour in the fkin of the abdomen, which becomes greenifh. There is no fimilar change in what is called the putrid fever. It may be alledged, that putrefaction is a different thing in the living, and in the dead body. But if this be admitted, and putrefaction in a living and in a dead body are allowed to be different proceffes, inferences drawn from

one

one can never be applied to the other, and the greater part, if not all, of the reafoning adduced on this fubject, muft fall to the ground.

Were it to be granted, that the diffolved ftate of the blood was the effect of putrefaction, there would ftill be no good ground to infer, that it was the caufe of the fever. It is confiftent with reafon, that the magnitude or intenfity of the caufe, fhould be proportioned to the greatnefs of the effect. In all cafes, therefore, of the fever there fhould be fome marks of putrefaction, and a violent degree of the difeafe could not be fuppofed to exift without them; yet this is by no means agreeable to obfervation. In many of the worft cafes of fever, and which fuddenly prove fatal, there are no appearances of the blood being in a diffolved ftate, nor are there any other marks of putrefaction. How then can putrefaction be fuppofed to be the

the caufe of a difeafe, which often exifts in the moft violent degree, and frequently puts an end to life, without the fainteft traces of the exiftence of fuch a procefs?

If we examine more minutely into this fubject, it will appear, that the opinion of the putrid nature of the difeafe is founded on a vague analogy, which will not ftand the teft of experiment, or obfervation. The diffolved ftate of the blood has been confidered as the moft unequivocal mark of the prefence of putrefaction; but the diffolution of the blood in fcurvy has been found not to proceed from putrefaction, for fuch blood does not putrify fooner than any other, which it ought to do, if already in a putrid ftate, when taken out of the body *. If the diffolved ftate of the blood in fcurvy do not depend on putrefaction, there is little rea-

---

* Lind on the Scurvy.

son to suppose, that in fevers it is owing to that cause. The dissolution often takes place in the course of a few hours, which cannot be explained from any thing observed to happen in putrefaction, which is a process that goes on slowly and regularly. The offensive smell proceeding from the persons of the sick, which is believed to depend upon putrefaction, is very different from that which arises from dead subjects in a dissecting room, as will be readily admitted by any one that has had experience of both; yet they ought not to differ, if they both depended on the putrefaction of an animal body. But farther, it often happens that the dead bodies have so little of an offensive smell, that it has been matter of surprise to those that have opened them *. There appears indeed to be no foundation for believing, that

* See Mr. M'Colme's Dissections, which are given p. 200.

putrefaction

putrefaction is the caufe of the remittent fever, or of any of its fymptoms, either when in the mildeſt, or moſt violent form. The hypotheſis, though not productive of equal miſchief in the treatment of the diſeaſe, as a belief of its bilious nature, is neither of uſe in explaining the fymptoms, nor in the cure; befides, it gives riſe to fome ill-founded notions, one of the worſt of which is a belief, that as the fever is of a putrid nature, ſo it muſt be infectious.

There is hardly any part of the hiſtory of a difeafe, which it is of more conſequence to afcertain with accuracy, than its being of an infectious nature, or not. Upon this depends the propriety of the fteps that ſhould be taken, either to prevent it, or to root it out. It is productive of great miſchief to confider a difeafe as infectious, that really is not fo; it expofes fuch as labour under it to evils and inconveniences, which greatly aggravate their sufferings, and often deprive them of the necessary assistance. They are neglected, if not shunned; and at the time they require the greatest care and attention, they have the least. I have had occasion to observe that the remittent fever, whether with its usual or more uncommon symptoms, with the yellow colour of the eyes and skin or without them, was never found to be infectious. The strongest proofs of this, in my opinion, were to be met with in private families, where the son, the brother, or the husband, labouring under the worst fevers, were nursed with unremitting assiduity by the mother, the sister, or the wife, who never left the sick either by day or by night, yet without being infected. That such near relations should take upon them the office of a nurse, is matter of the highest commendation in a country, the diseases of which require to be watched with greater care and attention, than can be expected from a servant.

They

They are under no fears of the fever being infectious, and I never saw any reason to believe it to be so, either in private families, or in the military hospitals. There appears not to be any necessary connection between infection and putrefaction, even supposing putrefaction to exist in a living body; infectious diseases are not necessarily putrid, nor are diseases, supposed to be the most putrid, as the scurvy, in the smallest degree infectious. The operation of a cause, generally diffused, is often confounded with the effects of infection.

Some have attempted to explain the *phænomena* of fever, by deducing them from one or other of the symptoms. The appearances have been supposed to depend upon the cold fit, and a constriction, or spasm, of the blood-vessels of the skin: but in the remittent fever there is often no cold fit, and it happens frequently, that the sick have the most profuse sweats without any abatement of the symptoms. The use of emetics in small

small doses, with a view to remove the spasm from the vessels of the skin, by producing sickness, and thence a disposition to perspire, is evidently liable to the same objections, as when had recourse to for the purpose of procuring a discharge of bile. Though the intention be different, the effect is the same upon a stomach highly irritable from the nature of the disease, and thence easily thrown into violent contractions.

Some have alledged the cause of the fever to be seated in the stomach. It cannot be denied that, in general, that organ suffers as early, and in as violent a degree in fevers, as any other in the human body; but it must be a vain attempt, to seek for the cause in any one of the symptoms, when every function of the whole frame is deranged.

The voluntary, and involuntary motions are equally affected, as are also the senses, and operations of the mind. The muscular fibre cannot contract with its usual

usual force, and thence a general loss of strength; the motion of the heart is too quick, and often irregular; the respiration is interrupted with frequent sighings; the stomach loaths food, and is unable to digest it; and the bowels are either too slow, or irregular in their action. The secretions, as of the mucus that lines the mouth, the urine, and the sweat, all undergo a change. Vision is neither clear, nor distinct; objects dance before the eyes, and even the impression of light is painful. The hearing is either disagreeably acute and offended with all kind of impressions, or very dull. The taste is changed, what was sweet before is perhaps salt, and what was highly grateful is become nauseous. The sense of smelling is equally perverted. The touch no longer judges of the degree of heat with truth, and the distressing symptoms of restlessness and constant change of posture, are in part owing to a morbid sensibility of every part of the body.

The

The operations of the mind are no lefs deranged than thofe of the body. An exertion either of the memory or judgement is fatiguing and painful, and after a fhort continuance impracticable. Mental impreffions are indiftinct, or erroneous. The imagination is wild and confufed, and paints to itfelf a thoufand fcenes full of error and delufion; and that faculty, by which the mind diftinguifhes the objects that pafs in the imagination from the real impreffions, is weakened, fometimes deftroyed, and thence delirium, at one time like a fit of madnefs, at another like a waking dream. The fleep neither brings reft to the body, nor quiet to the mind; and after a time the whole faculties of the foul are overwhelmed by ftupor, and general infenfibility.

Such being the *phænomena* of fever, it is impoffible to derive the fymptoms from an affection of the brain and nervous

vous system; for we often find all the functions of the brain and nerves deranged by local causes, as in palsy, mania, and other diseases as much as in fevers, yet the motion of the heart, and operations of the stomach, go on as in health, with little variation. Again, the pulsations of the heart are often as quick and irregular as in fever, from diseases of the heart, and surrounding parts, as ossifications of the valves, and dropsies of the thorax; yet the other functions are but little deranged, and there is no fever. The same reasoning will apply to the stomach; the functions of which, from local diseases, as scirrhus, and cancer, are often as much affected, as in the remittent fever, yet without producing that disease.

If it should be asked what explanation can be given of the phænomena of fever, I am ready to acknowledge my own ignorance; yet as it is impossible to give due attention to the appearances of fever, without this question presenting itself to the mind, I will state shortly, what appears to be a proper mode of investigating the subject.

The cause of the remittent fever is evidently the exhalations of wet or marshy ground, which may be considered as a poison to the human body *. The examination of those exhalations is the first step in the inquiry. Simple moisture in the air is perfectly harmless, in so far certainly as relates to the remittent fever. Marshy ground is known to produce inflammable air, which is found to be fatal when breathed of a certain strength, but when mixed with common air, is not known to produce any mischief †. Were inflammable air the cause of fevers, they would be fre-

---

* Cullen's First Lines, vol. I. § lxxxiv, ci.
† Philof. Transf. vol. lxix. p. 337.

quent

quent in mines, which is not the cafe. Though the caufe of fevers is not found in the inflammable air, yet the offenfive fmell of marfhes is in a great meafure owing to it. This inveftigation muft be extremely delicate, but confidering the great progrefs that has lately been made in the examination of all kinds of air, or elaftic vapour, it is not to be defpaired of.

The next queftion is, how does the poifon gain admiffion into the body? It may be by the lungs in refpiration; by the abforbing veffels of the fkin; or, by adhering to the *fauces* in refpiration, it may be fwallowed with whatever is carried down into the ftomach.

Late experiments have fhewn, that there is a portion of the air which enters the lungs in infpiration, abforbed by the blood paffing through the blood-veffels*.

* Prieftley on Air, vol. iii. fect. 5.

This portion would appear to be chiefly, if not altogether, the dephlogisticated air, which constitutes about a fifth part of atmospheric air. This air therefore uniting with the blood and entering into the circulation, may carry along with it any poison diffused through the atmosphere. The lymphatic vessels in the lungs may, possibly, absorb any poison that is mixed with the air.

There are numerous proofs of fevers being occasioned by the absorption of poisons from the surface of the body. In mortifications of the lower extremities, the absorption of a poison has been traced by inflamed lymphatics, and consequent swelling of the glands in the groin, which have been followed by a fever of some days continuance. An elderly woman, with an old fore in her leg, was subject to fevers, which held her several days; they were preceded by pain and swelling in the groin of the side on which

which the fore was; and there were red lines obfervable on the fkin, running from the fore to the groin, the marks undoubtedly of the poifon paffing through the lymphatics. In fuch cafes there is an evident fource of the poifon; but I have met oftener than once with the fame fwelling in the groin, followed by a confiderable, fometimes a violent degree of fever, and the courfe of the poifon could be traced by the inflamed lymphatics to the leg, where, however, there was no fore. Similar cafes are, I doubt not, frequent; but the language of the fick is apt to miflead the inquirer, for in general they fay the fever has fallen into the leg, as if the affection of the leg were a confequence of the fever; whereas, the fwelling of the glands of the groin will be found to have preceded the fever, and indeed it is commonly the firft fymptom to which attention is paid. Some fevers of this kind are very violent, and begin

begin with severe rigors, which are followed by great heat, delirium, and other alarming symptoms; but what the poison is, I have not yet met with any case from which I could form a conjecture. Many more facts might be adduced to shew, that fevers often arise from the absorption of poisons from the surface of the body; it is probable that the plague is communicated in this way, and that the buboes are not critical, but traces of the route by which the poison gets into the circulation. It is possible, the great danger of catching a fever from getting wet by rain, an opinion universally prevalent in the West Indies, may in part be owing to the vapours, when condensed and passing through the air, carrying along with them the poison.

The loss of appetite and sickness at stomach, which are common in the beginning of fever, may give reason to suspect that the cause of fever is first conveyed

veyed into the stomach, being mixed with the saliva and the mucus that lines the fauces, and so swallowed; and this suspicion may appear to some to be confirmed, by the good effects of such medicines as evacuate the stomach and bowels, upon the first attack of fever.

The poison having got admission into the body, the laws that regulate its operations are next to be inquired into. The violence of it would appear to depend upon two circumstances, which are found to have great influence upon the operation of many other poisons; the quantity and virulence of the poison; and the body having been more or less habituated to it. The poison appears to be strongest as it rises from the ground, and becomes weaker as it is more diffused, and mixed with a larger proportion of air. Houses on the ground are more unhealthy than those that are elevated *. The

* Bontius, Med. Ind. cap. xii.

neighbourhood of marshes is also unhealthy, particularly such places as lie to leeward of them; and as you recede from the marsh there is less sickness, till at last you get beyond its sphere of action, and that at no great distance. Fort Augusta is seated on a bank of sand, behind it is an inlet of the sea, and beyond that a considerable extent of marshy ground. The land wind blows every night from the marshes towards the fort, and they are not in a direct line three miles distant, yet they are not productive of fevers. How much less than three miles might be sufficient to do away the noxious effects of the exhalations, I am not in possession of facts to determine. It is probable that the distance may be affected by various circumstances; as the extent of the marsh, or the disposition of the hills in the neighbourhood, which may confine as in a funnel the streams of air, and give them a particular direction.

After

After the human body has been expofed to the poifon, fometimes a longer, fometimes a fhorter period elapfes, before a fever is produced. The men on the watering fervice are not all taken ill at the fame time; fome fall fick the firft or fecond day, and others not till feveral days after they have ceafed to be expofed to the caufe of fever, by returning on board of fhip. The poifon, it would appear, may lie dormant fome time in the body, though it is difficult to determine accurately how long. Some have embarked on board of fhip in good health, and have been feized after ten or fourteen days with the remittent fever. Examples in this way have come to my knowledge, of the fever appearing three weeks after ceafing to be expofed to the caufe of it; how much greater the interval may be, I know no facts to determine. We may venture to lay it down as an axiom, that the poifon will be more

or

or less mischievous, as it is more or less concentrated; a property that is not found in what may be called specific poisons, as that of small pox, the venereal disease, and others.

The power of habit, in counteracting the effects of the poison, are universally acknowledged. New-comers is not only more subject to the disease, but in them it is of the worst kind. A first attack is called in common language a *seasoning*. In this respect it is like many other poisons, to which the human body gradually accommodates itself. Opium may be swallowed in large quantities by those accustomed to it. The same is true of ardent spirits, and of most, if not all the substances that produce intoxication. The negroes, who live in marshy parts of the country, afford the most striking example of the power of habit in resisting the poison; they are very little subject to the fever, and in them it is almost always slight.

In

In the expedition against Fort St. Juan, not one in twenty of the soldiers returned, whereas none of the negroes died of fevers.

Another circumstance before noticed deserves to be more particularly investigated, as it renders the poison both more certain, and more violent in its effects; that is, being exposed to it when fatigued by hard labour and long fasting. The poison gains admission more readily into the body, and produces immediately the worst kind of fever. It is in this way that soldiers suffer so much, on actual service, in the West Indies. The few cases of fever which proved fatal in 24 hours, that occurred to me, were all contracted in a similar manner. A soldier taken ill on a march, and under the necessity of walking five or six miles, has scarcely a chance of recovering; and if he do not expire on the way, seldom survives the completion of the march many hours. In a fatigued and exhausted

exhausted state of the body, the vessels on the surface both of the skin and lungs, probably come to be in an inhaling state, and thus give freer admission to the poison; and the quickened circulation of the blood conveys it more speedily, and more intimately, to the minutest vessels of the body.

The most important question, after the poison has gained admission into the human body, is; How does it produce the symptoms of the fever? Our ignorance of the animal economy absolutely precludes us, from giving any adequate answer to this question. But when we consider, that every function of the human frame is deranged; that the blood is often in a dissolved state, and that there is a total loss of strength, we may conclude, that the poison affects the principles of life in every part of the body; and in fact we find that parts of the body do actually mortify, and die. What the

of the REMITTENT FEVER.

the principles of life are, we cannot yet form a conjecture, and to push our inquiries further on that side, would afford no satisfaction.

The illustrations, that apply best to our subject, are borrowed from the operations of poisons. Sickness and vomiting are the first effects of most poisons, animal as well as vegetable, and also of morbid poisons [*], and are likewise common at the commencement of fever. It is true some poisons, if sufficiently concentrated, as the laurel-water, poison of the Ticunas, and others, produce convulsions, and almost instant death [†]: analogous to this, the remittent fever often begins in children with fits, and sometimes also in adults. The blood comes to be in a dissolved state from many poisons, as

---

[*] According to Mr. Hunter's distinction. Vid. Treat. Ven. Dif. p. 9.

[†] Fontana, sur les Poisons, vol. ii. p. 83, 125, 137.

that of the viper; and the same poison is known to produce a jaundice, preceded by great loss of strength, and sometimes fainting fits. Here then are several of the symptoms of the worst kind of remittent fever, particularly the jaundice. I do not know of any instance of the body having been examined after death, occasioned by the bite of a serpent; but when the bodies of those, who have died of the yellow fever, have been opened, if there were any morbid appearances, for often there were none, they consisted chiefly in the internal coats of the stomach and duodenum being in an inflamed state. The gall in the bladder and ducts is generally found ropy and viscid, as if it had stagnated for some time, though no cause of obstruction appear in the duct. It is probable that the inflammation in the coats of the duodenum and stomach, and the violent contractions they suffer from repeated vomiting and straining, may

may produce a spasm of the gall ducts, sufficient to interrupt the course of the bile *. That the *ductus communis* possesses naturally a power of contraction in an healthy state cannot be doubted, for, without such a contraction in some part of it, the bile could never regurgitate so, as to fill the gall-bladder. That jaundice may proceed from other causes, besides a stoppage to the flow of the bile by *calculi* or mechanical pressure, must be allowed, as an examination of the body after death has often shewn no such causes to exist †. In the body of a person who died of pulmonary consumption, I had lately occasion to observe some things not altogether foreign to the present subject. A few days before death, to the common

* Fontana, sur les Poisons. vol. i. part. 5. ch. 13. p. 69.

† Morgagni, de Sed. et Cauf. Morb. Ep. 53. § 16, 17. Ep. 37. § 10.—Sir John Pringle, Dif. of Army, Appendix, p. cxix. edit. 7th.

symptoms of the difeafe, was fuperadded a jaundice. The lungs were found difeafed in the ufual manner; there were adhefions to the pleura, tubercles, indurations, and fuppurations in their fubftance. In the abdomen there were marks of fuperficial inflammation all over the liver, and the lower furface of it was united to the ftomach by adhefions. The gallbladder was full, but no bile could be fqueezed out of it. On laying the *ductus communis* open from the *duodenum*, it was found filled with bile of a brown colour, and of a thick and ropy confiftence, as were alfo the *ductus hepatici*. Part of the *ductus cyfticus* was laid open, and the gallbladder was preffed with confiderable force, but ftill no bile flowed. Through a blow-pipe introduced into the duct, the air at laft with fome difficulty was forced into the gall-bladder, after which by preffing again, a coagulum of bile was fqueezed out, and what followed was ropy

ropy and black, like melasses. On laying the duct open all the way to the bladder, there appeared no other obstruction to the bile than the coagulum, which, as well as the thick and ropy state of that secretion, appear rather to have been the effects of stagnation, than a cause of obstruction in the first instance. Did the inflammation in the neighbourhood of the ducts, and perhaps extending to them, excite such contractions in them as obstructed the bile, in the same way that a suppression of urine, is sometimes a consequence of inflammation, in the urinary passages?

The cause of the jaundice, in the remittent fever, deserves to be farther investigated in the dead body, and I have to regret that I did not attend to it more while in Jamaica. The following letter, containing an account of the dissections of 23 bodies, was written to the late Sir John Pringle by Mr. John M'Colme, a man of veracity and obfervation, who ferved as a regimental furgeon in the Weſt Indies, in the years 1741 and 1742.

ANATOMICAL FACTS *from the opened Bodies of* 23 *Officers and Soldiers, who died of the Bilious, or Yellow Fever, in the Weſt Indies.*

"IN all the cafes the liver was
"changed in part (and fometimes almoſt
"the whole) to be more pale, and hard,
"than natural; and in fuch parts there
"was a lefs proportion of blood, than
"in thofe of a more natural colour.

"In fuch as greatly differed in colour
"and hardnefs, there were found obftruc-
"tions in the larger branches of the
"vena porta, refembling what are called
"*polypi.*

"The bile in the gall-bladder, of a
"deeper colour, much thicker and more
"vifcous,

" viscous, than common; small in quan-
" tity, never exceeding an ounce; oftener
" from half an ounce to six drachms.

" The spleen larger, softer, and whiter,
" than common.

" The internal part of the stomach
" and duodenum sometimes reddish, or
" yellow, but often blackish; the tu-
" nica villosa very easily separating, even
" with the touch; the other guts much
" in the same state: but in general the
" two first most affected.

" In the stomach often a thick mucus,
" with the same black stuff that is
" thrown up by vomit: if the villous
" coat is not much affected, the mucus
" prevails; but if otherwise the *black*
" *vomit*.

" Farther down the guts the black
" stuff is thicker, and more viscid, al-
" most resembling tar; and in the great
" guts it is often mixed with clotted
" blood.

" The cellular and other membranes
" much

"much diftended with blood; the ten-
"dinous part of the diaphragm and
"pleura look as if injected.

"In one perfon who had been troubled
"with a violent hickup, there was an
"ulcer on the tendinous part of the dia-
"phragm, that difcharged fanies into the
"thorax.

"The lungs were often blackifh next
"the pleura, and interfperfed in many
"places with large livid fpots.

"In the right ventricle of the heart,
"*finus venofus*, and *vena cava*, there
"was lefs blood than common.

"The urine in the bladder common-
"ly yellow.

"One thing was remarkable, that
"notwithftanding the bodies both be-
"fore, and after death, had a very dif-
"agreeable ftench; yet upon opening
"the abdomen and the guts, there was
"not near fo cadaverous or fœtid a
"fmell, as there is generally in Europe.
"They

"They were indeed opened foon after death; and generally had been purged during their illnefs.

"It is worth while to obferve, that two bodies were alfo opened; each of which formerly had the bilious fever; but died fome time after from other caufes. None of them had obftructions in the liver, and the bile in the gall-bladder was larger in quantity, and more fluid than common.

"All thefe bodies were opened by the direction of Dr. Robert Dalrymple, phyfician to the army, in the years 1741, 1742. At the opening of many of them I was prefent; the reft the doctor told me were fimilar to what I faw."

The morbid appearances mentioned in the letter, are nearly all referable to two caufes; the abforption of the bile into the general mafs of circulating fluids, and

and more or less of a dissolution of the blood. The pale colour of the liver and spleen, depended on the bile that had been absorbed, and mixed with the blood; under which circumstances it tinges those *viscera,* and almost every part of the body, of a yellow colour, as is seen in common cases of jaundice. The black matter, found in the stomach and bowels, appears evidently to have been the blood, that had oozed through the vessels; and this, as well as the livid spots upon the lungs, are proofs of the dissolved state of the blood. Similar livid spots are often found upon the lungs of animals that die of poisons, and proceed from the blood being in a dissolved state *.

Though a comparison of the effects of other poisons with those of the exhalations of marshes, promises to throw more light on the subject of the remittent fever,

* Vid. Fontana, sur les Poisons. vol. i. part. 3. chap. 3.

than any other mode of inveftigation that prefents itfelf, yet the inquiry cannot be pufhed a great way. There is fomething uncommonly fubtle and abftrufe in the operations of poifons, as may be deduced from this, that of the various poifons of which we have daily experience, there is none of whofe effects we can give any good explanation. Moft of the morbid poifons are confined to one fpecies of animals, yet we can fee nothing in the poifon, or in the fpecies, to account for this. The fmall-pox, meafles, plague, and many other difeafes affect the human fpecies only, though no reafon appears why it fhould be fo; and any explanation of thofe difeafes, whether derived from fermentation, putrefaction, or a peculiar action of veffels, contains nothing to inftruct us, why they fhould not affect other animals as well as man. Putrefaction is the fame nearly in all animal matter; and we have not yet learnt from phyfiology

logy or anatomy, any peculiar properties or actions that our blood-veſſels poſſeſs, which are not to be found in many other animals. But although the inveſtigation of the operation of poiſons on animal bodies be a ſubject of extreme difficulty, it is not to be deſpaired of; nor are we, in any caſe, to ſet limits and boundaries to the advancement of human knowledge, by experiment and obſervation.

Sect. IV. *Of Intermittent Fevers.*

INTERMITTENT fevers, as quotidians, tertians, quartans, and all the variations of them uſually mentioned by writers, occur frequently in Jamaica. The fevers that prevail moſt, during the more healthy part of the year, are intermittents; whereas, during the rains, and for ſome time after,

Of Intermittent Fevers.

after, they are chiefly remittents: as if both depended upon the same cause, acting at different times with more or less violence. The almost endless varieties of intermittent fevers, described by the ancients, have ceased in a great measure to be the objects of attention, since the Peruvian bark has been discovered, to be the most efficacious remedy against them all, whatever type they assume. While it was believed, that the various forms of the disease required peculiar modes of treatment, it was deemed a matter of the last consequence to distinguish them rightly.

In the history of intermittent fevers in Jamaica, there is little to be observed that is peculiar to the climate. The cold fit is generally less severe than in more northern latitudes, and during its continuance it is not uncommon for the sick, to expose themselves to the direct rays of the sun, taking in this an example from the negroes, who thereby more effectually

relieve

relieve the painful sensations of cold, than by sitting over the fire, or covering the body with a load of bed-clothes, as practised in colder countries.

The quotidian is the most dangerous form of the disease, and is more or less so, as it approaches to, or recedes from, a remittent fever. The tertian is less dangerous, and the quartan least of all; though there, as well as in other countries, it is extremely obstinate and difficult of cure.

Sect. V. *Of the Cure of Intermittent Fevers.*

WHEN the intermissions were compleat, the bark was given directly, without any previous evacuations, in order to cleanse the stomach and bowels,

els, which is to be confidered as rather recurring to an old, than giving into a new practice *. There was no inconvenience arofe from omitting the vomiting and purging, ufually made to precede the bark; on the contrary it was fo much time gained. The bark was given in the dofe of one or two drachms in wine, or any other vehicle that was more agreeable to the fick, and repeated every two hours, or oftener, according to the urgency of the cafe, and the ftate of the ftomach.

After the progrefs of the difeafe was ftopped, it was ftill proper to give a dofe of the bark twice or thrice a day, for five or fix days, in order to prevent a relapfe. If the bark rendered the body coftive, half an ounce of the tincture of fena, or of rhubarb, or an aloetic pill was given at bed-time; or a few grains of rhubarb

* Vid. Sydenham, Proceffus integri, de Feb. Intermitt.

were added to one or more doses of the bark.

Although the bark be not less efficacious in the cure of intermittents in Jamaica, than in other parts of the world, yet it happened that there were cases which did not yield to it, though given liberally, and for a length of time. In such cases various means were tried, and to some of them the fever commonly gave way; although it was difficult to determine to which a preference was due, as sometimes one appeared more successful, sometimes another. Chamomile flowers reduced to a fine powder, and given in the dose of half a drachm, or even a drachm, and repeated every three hours, often stopt the fever after the bark had failed. A warm purgative, as six drachms of the tincture of rhubarb, and as much of the tincture of sena, was sometimes given six or seven hours before the fit, and the bark as usual, after it was

over

over. This as well as the chamomile flowers sometimes failed, and sometimes succeeded.

The cold bath, in the river at Spanish Town, was effectual in subduing old intermittents in many instances. The bath was taken in the morning, when the temperature of the river might be from 75° to 80°.

Sal ammoniac, or alum, were sometimes added to the bark, and the former was given in some instances by itself, but their power did not appear great, though they stopped the fever in some cases.

For some years past, intermittents have been more frequent in, and about London, than formerly. Since my return from Jamaica, I have often joined mercurials * to the bark in the treatment of such fevers, when they have proved obstinate, and with good success. The preparation made use of was the *mercurius dulcis*,

* Vid. Med. Transf. Vol. III.

which

which was sometimes given in the quantity of 3 or 4 grains along with 15 or 20 grains of jalap, so as to prove purgative; but more commonly in smaller doses, and by itself at bed-time, so as to keep the body only moderately open. For this purpose one or two grains every night, or every other night according to circumstances, were generally sufficient, while the bark was given in the usual way, during the intermissions of the fever. The mercurial gave new efficacy to the bark, and this treatment often proved successful. It is probable a similar practice might succeed in the West Indies, though I have no experience of it.

Towards the end of the war some red bark was sent to Jamaica, which given in the same dose with the common bark affected the bowels, producing sickness and vomiting, or griping, purging and flatulence. The dose was therefore restricted to half a drachm, which was repeated

peated every three hours, and cured many intermittents that had refifted the common bark. The great tendency which it had to affect the ftomach and bowels, rendered it lefs proper than the common bark in the remittent fever, and on that account, after a few trials, it was laid afide in that fpecies of the difeafe. Whether it would have been more efficacious in curing intermittents, if given in the firft inftance, than common bark, is a queftion that I had not an opportunity of bringing to a fair decifion; for though it often cured fevers that refifted the common bark, yet nearly as much might be faid of the chamomile flowers, though that would not be good ground for fuppofing the latter medicine a better than the former. If the red bark, and the common bark, were given in the firft inftance in a number of intermittents, that would doubtlefs be deemed the beft medicine, which cured the greatest proportion of the sick. In order to form a just judgment, the number of cases ought to be considerable, certainly not less than ten for each of the medicines. Simple as this experiment is, I do not know that it has yet been tried. In the mean time we may safely conclude, that we are in possession of a valuable medicine, which will often succeed, after the common bark has failed.

It has been already observed, that the remittent fever, after repeated attacks, often produces dropsy, or swellings of the liver or spleen, and frequently a complication of both these disorders; the same thing holds true of intermittents. Those labouring under such accumulated distempers, are hardly to be restored by any means that can be employed, while they remain upon the island. The constitution, broken down in every part, can only be repaired by having recourse to a colder

Intermittent Fevers. 215

colder climate, and a more salubrious air; and even these are often deferred till it be too late. The air of the mountains, and a frequent change of it in travelling by easy journeys, together with bitters to strengthen the stomach, and occasionally small doses of mercurials, will often procure a temporary amendment. The mercurial given for the swellings of the liver or spleen, was the mercurius dulcis, which was exhibited in small doses. In cases of dropsy, quicksilver, rubbed down with an equal quantity of honey or conserve of hips, was given; the dose was from five to ten grains of the mass, to which half a grain, or even a whole grain of the dried squills was added, to render it diuretic; and it was repeated every other night for ten days, or a longer or shorter time, according to circumstances. If advantage, however, were not taken of any favourable change in the health, from the means just mentioned, the disease generally recurred in a short time with greater violence, and soon proved fatal.

CHAP.

CHAP. IV.

Of the DYSENTERY.

SECT. I. *Of the Symptoms of the Dysentery.*

IN treating of the dysentery, I have confined myself to such observations, as more particularly apply to the climate, or have not hitherto been made; not judging it necessary to enter minutely either into the history of the disease, or the method of cure, which have been so fully treated by much abler hands.

The dysentery, as it appears in the island of Jamaica, is the same disease that is so well described by Sydenham,

Sir

Sir John Pringle, Sir George Baker, and others; and is not diſtinguiſhed by any peculiar ſymptoms from the dyſentery, that was epidemic in London, in the ſummer and autumn of the years 1779, and 1780.

There ſubſiſts an intimate connection between the remittent fever and this diſeaſe, in Jamaica; the one frequently changes into the other, and the two diſeaſes are often complicated with various degrees of violence. In ſome caſes the dyſentery ends in a fever, though it happens much oftener that the fever terminates in a dyſentery, eſpecially among the common ſoldiers.

In ſome ſeaſons the dyſentery is much more frequent than in others, which was the caſe in 1782; the cauſe of this is not ſo obvious. It was hotter than common in the month of June by three or four degrees, the thermometer riſing many days to 90°, an unuſual heat in that climate,

climate. An higher degree of heat than common, in our summers in England, has been observed to be productive of dysenteries, as was the case in the summers above mentioned; but, in Jamaica, the coolest month in the year is at least $12°$ hotter, than the hottest month in our summers: if the cause therefore depended upon any absolute degree of heat, the dysentery should prevail all the year round. How far it may arise from a comparative increase merely in the heat, though there is some ground to suspect it may be so, I have not sufficient experience to determine.

There are various degrees of violence in the disease, from slight gripings with frequent slimy stools, to the most excruciating pains in the bowels, incessant straining, profuse discharge of blood, great fever, and sudden prostration of strength. Between these extremes are numerous intermediate degrees, and though

though the flighter cafes may be called by the name of diarrhœa, yet there are no specific marks of diftinction; they run into one another by an infenfible gradation, and therefore should not be diftinguished by different names *.

There are some of the quarters, such as Fort Augufta, and Port Royal, fubject to a mild kind of dyfentery, especially when the foldiers firft take poffeffion of them. It is probably owing to the water in both places, for as they are situated upon fand-banks nearly furrounded by the fea, they have no freth water but what is brought to them, commonly from the mouth of the Spanifh Town river. This

---

* The antients apply the terms Dyfentery, Diarrhœa, Lienteria, Tenefmus, &c. to the feveral ftages or fymptoms of this difeafe, and confider them as feparate and diftinct diftempers. Some of the fymptoms of fever they have alfo treated as diftinct difeafes, as phrenitis, and lethargus, which are the delirious and comatofe ftages of fever. Vid. Cœl. Aurelian.

water

water becomes extremely putrid, especially if put in casks that formerly contained rum, and in such a state is undoubtedly hurtful to the bowels. There are other circumstances in the management of the water, that deserve to be noticed; it is sometimes kept in cisterns, in which millions of insects, particularly musquitoes, breed; the negroes likewise employed in taking up the water, do not always proceed far enough from the mouth of the river, to get clear of all admixture of salt water, so that it is sometimes brackish. That such water should produce complaints of the bowels, will not appear surprising, and it is probably the sole cause of them *. Yet, it were to be wished that Fort Augusta, and Port Royal were supplied with good water, such as that of the watering-place for the royal navy, and that it were kept in

---

* Bontius de Med. Ind. dialog. 3^{tio}.

proper casks: for, by these means it would be ascertained beyond a doubt, what share the water had in producing the flux.

A symptom that frequently occurs in the disease, and is not taken notice of by the authors above quoted, is an immediate call to go to stool, upon swallowing any thing either solid or liquid, accompanied with a feeling, as if what was just swallowed, were running through the bowels. This sensation is often so strong, that the sick imagine that the food they have taken has really passed through them, and are not convinced of the contrary, till they find that the discharge has been slime or mucus, without any resemblance to what they had swallowed. This symptom shews great irritability in the bowels, by which a motion excited in the stomach, is propagated almost directly to the anus.

The dysentery did not appear to be infectious

infectious in the hofpitals in Jamaica, nor in the epidemic that prevailed in London in the years 1779 and 1780. I am far from meaning to fay, that the dyfentery is never infectious; but there is fome difficulty in determining a queftion of this kind, for unlefs the proofs of infection are clear and decided, they may be eafily confounded with the effects of a caufe, that is generally diffufed, and operating upon all more or lefs, fuch as the caufe of dyfentery muft be.

SECT. II. *Of the Cure of the Dyfentery.*

THE dyfentery, like the fever, requires to be taken care of early, for the means that will either overcome, or greatly mitigate the difeafe at the beginning, will not be able to make any impreffion upon it, after it has continued fome some time. The first medicine that was given was a purgative. The kind of purgative most commonly made use of was the bitter purging salt *, or Glauber's salt †, sometimes with manna, and always with one or two drops of the oil of peppermint, added to the solution of the salt. An ounce of salt, and half that quantity of manna, dissolved in half a pint of water, with the addition of the oil of peppermint, were divided into two parts, which were given with an interval of half an hour or a whole hour between them, according to the state of the stomach. The operation of the physic is promoted by drinking plentifully of thin water-gruel, whey, chicken water, tea, or any diluting liquor that is most agreeable to the sick. In this way several copious stools are procured, whereby the

---

* Magnesia Vitriolata, Pharm. Lond. 1788.
† Natron Vitriolatum, Pharm. Lond. 1788.

griping

griping and other symptoms are greatly relieved. After a favourable operation of the physic, an opiate, from fifteen to twenty drops of the tinctura thebaica, was given at bed-time. The purgative in almost all cases procures a truce with the disease, and the opiate prolongs it.

It is in slight cases only, and at the commencement of the disease, that one dose of physic is sufficient to stop its progress; a respite merely is in general all that is obtained. When the symptoms recur, the same medicines are to be repeated. The sick are not weakened by the operation of the purgatives, at least as long as they procure relief from the griping pain. When the disease is violent however, and the purgatives have been frequently repeated, and the symptoms still recur at the same time that the strength is greatly impaired, there is a period beyond which purgatives cannot be longer given with advantage. In this

this situation I have repeatedly made use of the following medicine with great benefit; two table spoonfuls of a strong decoction or infusion of the bark, and the same quantity of strong chamomile tea, were made into a draught, to which as much rhubarb was added, as would procure two or three copious discharges from the bowels in the twenty-four hours. The quantity of rhubarb usually added was about five grains, the draughts were given every three hours, and the rhubarb was either increased, diminished, or altogether omitted according to its operation. It may deserve to be noticed, that the sick can readily distinguish the motions proceeding from the disease, from those produced by a purgative medicine. I first gave this medicine in cases where there was a considerable degree of fever, together with the dysenteric symptoms; but I have since given it, and with good effect, when there has been little or no fever,

fever, but the strength of the patient has been too much reduced to bear purgatives.

The griping pains of the bowels, which are often excruciating, are relieved by fomentations applied to the abdomen, and still more effectually by blisters on the same part.

It is sometimes impossible to begin the cure with a purgative, owing to great sickness at stomach and vomiting. Under such circumstances, the evacuation of the stomach is promoted by giving warm water, or weak chamomile tea; and nothing more powerfully emetic is administered. As soon as the stomach is quieted, one or two drachms of the purging salts are given at a time, and repeated every hour, till they have had the desired effect. The treatment is afterwards the same as mentioned above.

After getting over the first attack, the chronic stage of the disease often follows.

This confifts of frequent returns of the griping, ftraining, and purging, with fhort intervals of eafe. The intervals feldom exceed one or two days; the ftrength and flefh wafte, hectic fever comes on, and more perifh in this ftage of the diforder than by the firft attack. The remedies here are nearly the fame as thofe above mentioned; nothing procures equal relief with a medicine gently opening, and the opiate muft now be given more freely; the ufe of it indeed can hardly be difpenfed with for one night. It may appear liable to objection to give an opening medicine at a period of the difeafe, which is fuppofed to depend upon a laxity of the bowels, and to require aftringents. That the chronic ftage of the difeafe may fometimes proceed from a mere laxity, I have no doubt; but fuch cafes are neither very frequent, nor, I apprehend, dangerous. Nine out of ten, at leaft, of the chronic dyfenteries dysenteries depend upon obstructions, and a diseased state of the bowels, as the dissection of the dead bodies demonstrates. The morbid appearances of the bowels, after death, throw great light on the disease, I shall therefore mention them shortly.

Upon a first view the bowels particularly the colon, appear irregularly contracted, and redder than natural at the contracted parts. Upon a nearer inspection, by cutting out portions of the gut and examining the internal coats, the appearances of disease become more evident. There are to be seen small tubercles, like pustules, sometimes in a smaller, sometimes in a greater number; and they are to be found in different stages, so that their progress can only be collected from several observations combined. The same subject will frequently furnish, in different portions of the gut, examples of the several stages. Their progress appears to be nearly as follows; there is first a small round tubercle of a reddish colour, and not more than one tenth of an inch in diameter; it increases gradually till it be near a quarter of an inch in diameter, and becomes paler as it grows larger. In this stage there appears a small crack on the top with a slight depression, which gradually increase; and on examining the contents of the little tumour, I have generally found them to be a cheese-like substance. The pustule, for though it contain no *pus*, I do not know any name more expressive of its appearance, is seated under the villous coat, between that and the muscular coat. As the opening enlarges, the edges become prominent, and the base grows rough and scabrous, from which matter oozes out, that is sometimes tinged with blood. Such is the progress of one, but they are often in clusters, and become confluent,

ent, so as to form a rough unequal ulcerated surface, with an hard and thickened base. Sometimes they appear like a small eating ulcer in the gut, in which the prominence of the edges give an appearance of a loss of substance, or as if the villous coat were intirely removed.

These morbid appearances probably take place more or less, in all cases of epidemic dysentery. They were first taken notice of, as far as I know, by Mr. Hewson *, and afterwards by Dr. Woollaston †. Whether they are constant and invariable, remains to be determined by future observations: they were found in all the dysenteric subjects that I have examined, but that number is not considerable, and we are not warranted to conclude, that there may not be va-

---

* Vid. Pringle, Dis. of Army, ed. 7th. p. 243. p. iii. ch. 6. § 2.
† Baker's Libellus de Cat. & Dys. sub finem.

rious morbid appearances, peculiar to the difeafe under different circumftances. Sir John Pringle has indeed mentioned mortifications, gangrene, and abrafions of the villous coat, none of which I have ever feen; and there is reafon to fufpect, that the black colour arifing from extravafated blood has been taken for mortification, or beginning gangrene, which I the more readily mention, that the learned author acquainted me in his lifetime, that he put but little confidence in any of the diffections of dyfenteric patients, which were made in the military hofpitals, as the bowels were not infpected minutely. Sentiments, not much different from thefe, are to be found in his book *. The tubercles are moft frequently found in the great guts, but they are alfo fometimes to be met with in the *ileum*; and there is an appearance

---

* Page 250, 7th. ed.

of more or lefs of inflammation in their neighbourhood. It is perhaps unneceffary to mention, that the tubercles with their various ftages cannot be obferved without wafhing off the mucus, blood, and matter, that cover the inner furface of the gut.

Several of the fymptoms may be illuftrated from the morbid ftate of the parts, as they appear upon diffection. The fmall grains of cheefe-like matter often voided by the fick, moft probably proceed from the tubercles upon their firft opening; the thin watery ftools, with a mixture of blood, like the *lotura carnium*, arife from the ferum difcharged from the numerous little ulcers; and if the blood be in a diffolved ftate, or the inflammation great, much red blood may ooze out, and give the evacuations the appearance of confifting almoft entirely of blood. When the difeafe is violent, it is probable that the whole furface of the gut may be covered with

with tubercles; in which cafe great inflammation joined to violent fpafms and contractions of the bowels, excited by fo many irritating caufes, muft foon prove fatal. Should however the fick have ftrength to bear up againft the firft attack of the difeafe, they will often have to ftruggle againft the evils arifing from numerous fmall ulcers in the bowels, the confequences of the tubercles, which bring on what has been called the chronic ftage.

The tubercles and confequent fmall ulcers, when in clufters, occafion a confiderable contraction of the paffage, not fo much by their projecting into the cavity, as by the fpafms they excite in the mufcular coats of the gut. The diminution of the canal obftructs in part the paffage of the contents of the bowels, which accumulating muft at laft be propelled by greater efforts, and when forced through the contracted parts they occafion pain, griping,

griping, and frequent calls to go to stool, which recur from time to time, and characterise the chronic stage of the disease. It is also accompanied in general by an hectic fever, proceeding from an absorption of matter from the tubercles or little ulcers; for it deserves to be remarked, that the glands in that part of the mesentery, which corresponds with the diseased gut, are not in a sound state, but much enlarged and of a softer texture than natural.

In the chronic stage, laxatives rather than purgatives are to be used, as the sick have not strength to bear a strong medicine, though they require the passage to be kept open. Two or three drachms of the purging salts will often have the desired effect, or a few grains of rhubarb, or a spoonful of the *oleum ricini*. The opiate must be repeated after their operation, and indeed it will commonly be necessary to give it every night.

A light

A light nourishing diet, consisting chiefly of milk, broths, and gruels, contributes to the cure.

When the stools are frequent and copious, and without griping or pain, astringents may be used with advantage; but such cases are not very numerous. The extract of the *lignum Campechense*, is a good astringent in such cases, as are also the *cortex granati*, and *terra Japonica* *. One of these will sometimes succeed after another has failed, though I have not learned what the particular cases are to which they are peculiarly adapted. I have generally made trial of them in the order in which they are mentioned.

If the disease terminate in a *tenesmus*, or if that symptom prove troublesome, it is often entirely removed, and always greatly relieved, by an anodyne clyster

* More properly *catechu*. Pharm. Lond. 1788.

consisting of thirty or forty drops of the tinctura thebaica in three or four ounces of linseed tea, or a thin jelly of starch. SYDENHAM leaves this symptom to itself, though it is often extremely troublesome.

I shall conclude the subject of dysentery, with some observations on the remedies usually employed against that disease.

Blood-letting has been strongly recommended by some, and condemned by others. The appearance of inflammation in the bowels on dissection, would seem to shew the propriety of that evacuation. Yet it must be allowed that there may be an inflammation, that is, redness, swelling, and pain in a part, for which it would be highly improper to let blood, as is the case in all erysipelatous inflammations. The question, however, can only be determined by experience; and all that I have learned on the subject

amounts

amounts to this, that in flighter cafes, or when the difeafe is treated early, purgatives have proved fo effectual, that I have never had recourfe to bleeding: and when the difeafe has been more violent, the ftrength of the patient has been fo much reduced of a fudden, that I have not dared to make ufe of that evacuation. Poffibly there may be circumftances under which it would not only be fafe but highly advantageous, and it were to be wifhed thefe were accurately afcertained.

Vomits are ftrongly recommended in this difeafe, and it has been common to give them as the firft ftep in the cure. The fick are generally relieved by them, but the benefit is not fo great as that derived from a purgative, which is both more eafy and more effectual in its operation. The ficknefs produced by an emetic is often very diftreffing, and it is moft beneficial when it proves purgative. Upon thefe grounds therefore recourfe course was had in the first instance to the purgative, as the more certain and speedy means of procuring relief.

There are various purgatives recommended by different authors. The bitter purging salt *, or Glauber's salt †, as mentioned before, were found the best. They operated easily, speedily, and effectually. It is probable there is nothing specific in any purgative, and that they are more or less beneficial, as they possess in a greater or less degree, the properties just mentioned. Rhubarb and calomel, infusion of sena, castor oil, soluble tartar ‡, or any other purgative, may be given that experience has shewn to agree with particular constitutions.

There is scarcely any part of the practice concerning which authors are more divided, than in the use of opiates against the

---

* Magnesia vitriolata. Pharm. Lond. 1788.
† Natron vitriolatum. Pharm. Lond. 1788.
‡ Kali tartarisatum. Pharm. Lond. 1788.

dysentery.

dysentery. Sydenham in many cases is disposed to trust the cure entirely to them, while others of almost equal authority, condemn them universally in this disease. Sir John Pringle recommends them strongly, with this precaution, that they should not be given till a free evacuation has been procured by a purgative. In his manner of treating the disease, an opiate cannot be given till the end of the second day, as the first is employed in giving an emetic. In the method recommended above, an opiate is given in ten or twelve hours, or as soon as the purgative has operated freely. If the griping and other symptoms are relieved by the physic, an opiate never fails to do good by prolonging the truce thus obtained with the disease; but if no relief be obtained, which however never happens except in the very worst cases, the opiate does little or no good. It is objected that the truce obtained by the opiate is fallacious,

fallacious, and of short continuance. That the disease commonly recurs, except in the slighter cases, must be admitted, but this cannot be laid to the charge of the opiate, which considerably retards its return: and if any objection is to be made to the use of this medicine, it should be that it is not able so completely to subdue the disease, that it shall not return. But although neither that, nor any other medicine we are yet acquainted with, possess a virtue so much to be wished for, it is still of great importance, in a disease that so severely harrasses and debilitates the sick, to procure even a temporary relief to their sufferings, whereby they are better enabled to bear the operation of medicines afterwards necessary, and to support themselves against the disease.

Opiates were sometimes combined with an emetic or purgative medicine, as ipecacuanha, emetic tartar, or rhubarb;

barb; and this practice had often good effects in the chronic stage: but upon the whole I preferred their alternate use to combining them; as the emetic, if in sufficient quantity to produce sensible effects, occasioned a distressing nausea, and the opiate too much checked the effects of the purgative. It did not appear of much consequence, whether the opiate was given in a liquid, or a solid form. In some cases the Dover's powder*, in the dose of ten or fifteen grains, had good effects. It happened in this disease, as in others where opiates are given, that the head or stomach were sometimes disagreeably affected by them the next day. To obviate this various means were tried, none of which succeeded so well, as giving one or two spoonfuls of lemon-juice along with the opiate, though that often failed.

* Pulvis ipecacuanhæ comp. Pharm. Lond. 1788.

CHAP.

CHAP. V.

Of the Colic, or Dry-Belly-Ach.

SECT. I. *Of the Symptoms of the Dry-Belly-Ach.*

THE dry-belly-ach was formerly much more frequent in Jamaica, than it is at present. It is not confined to any particular season of the year, but prevails sometimes in one, sometimes in another; and at such times it cannot be said to be epidemic, as it is frequently confined to one place, and to persons of a particular description. In the months of April, May, and June, 1781, it was very frequent among the men of the

92d regiment at Spanish Town, while the better sort of the inhabitants were not at all affected by it. In the year following, there was occasion to make the same observation at Kingston, where the colic was prevalent among the private men of the 79th regiment. It proceeded from a cause, whose operation was confined almost entirely to the common soldiers, and which affected in an inconsiderable degree the lower class of inhabitants.

The disease began with slight uneasiness in the bowels, which was soon followed by great pain, accompanied with dejection, anxiety, and restlessness. The pain was of a dull kind, and generally confined to one part of the abdomen, which distinguished it from gripings of the bowels. It was aggravated by pressure on the part more immediately affected, though the sick sometimes thought themselves relieved by a general compression preffion of the abdomen. After a time the pain increafed, and often became excruciating, in fo much that men of great refolution could not lie quiet a moment, but were conftantly rolling about, and complaining even aloud of their fufferings. Nature indeed feemed unable to fupport the torments of the difeafe, and there were many inftances of the fick falling into ftrong convulfions, and epileptic fits, and of their remaining in a ftate of total infenfibility for many hours. After the pain had continued fome time, ficknefs at ftomach generally came on, together with vomiting and violent retchings; a glafs of water, in fome cafes, would not remain even a few minutes upon the ftomach.

The pulfe was not quicker than natural, nor was there any heat upon the fkin at the beginning of the complaint; but in its progrefs the pulfe generally became more frequent, which appeared to proceed

proceed more from the pain and sufferings of the sick, than the presence of fever. During the whole of the disease there prevailed a most obstinate constipation of the bowels, and there was often more or less of strangury. The duration, and also violence of the symptoms, admitted of great variety; but as means of relief were immediately had recourse to, and the disease was not allowed to run its course, it is not so easy to say what its natural progress would have been. The strength of the disease was broken as soon as a free passage could be obtained. In some cases this was effected in the course of twenty-four hours, though more commonly not before the end of the second or third day; and in some instances, where the disease was very bad, it was the tenth or eleventh day before evacuations were procured.

 Those, who have once had the disease,
remain

remain liable to relapfes, which are generally more violent than the firft attack; and their recovery becomes every time more flow, and lefs complete. The ftrength decays, the flefh waftes, particularly the mufcles of the arms, and in a moft remarkable degree the ball of the thumb; the complexion becomes pale and fallow, and the countenance expreffive of much dejection. In this ftate, and commonly after a fecond or third attack of the colic, they become paralytic.

The palfy may be confidered as the fecond ftage of the difeafe. It feldom follows the firft attack of colic, and not often the fecond, unlefs it has been violent; but few efcape more or lefs of it after a third, or fourth fit. The palfy comes on as the pain of the bowels abates; the fick complain of pain and forenefs in the arms, efpecially about the wrifts, and they find themfelves unable to move the arms, and particularly to perform those motions that depend upon the wrist. This is the slightest degree of palsy, but it is often more severe, and the sick cannot move either the arms, hands, or fingers. The palsy is most commonly confined to the upper extremities, though there are numerous examples of the lower being affected also: there are not indeed wanting instances of an almost total palsy, which followed some colics of unusual violence, and long duration. The sick lay on their back without motion in their legs or arms, with little or no power over the muscles of the neck and head, with a voice no louder than a whisper, and in two cases to these symptoms was superadded almost a total loss of sight, and hearing. Their recovery from such a situation is always extremely slow, and often incomplete; yet there were few to whom the disease proved fatal; for of several hundreds

dreds that were ill not more than four or five died, and thofe were not in the paralytic ftage of the difeafe, but in the convulfions and fits produced by the colic. Yet, though few died, many were loft to the fervice; for fome never recovered the ufe of their wrifts at all, and many more never acquired any ftrength either in their wrifts or arms, and became of courfe unfit for foldiers.

It muft be obvious, that in giving this fhort defcription of the colic, that was prevalent among the foldiers at Kingfton, and Spanifh Town, I have been defcribing a difeafe exactly fimilar in its fymptoms, progrefs, and confequences, to the *colica pictonum*, or painter's colic; and I might perhaps with propriety have referred to the full defcriptions, and accurate accounts of this difeafe, which have been publifhed by fome able and learned authors [*]; but I was willing to enable

[*] Vid. Med. Tranf. vol. ii. p. 68.—vol. iii. p. 407.

every one, by a short history of the dry-belly-ach, to draw his own conclusions respecting the identity of the two diseases.

SECT. II. *Of the Cure of the Dry-Belly-Ach.*

THE principal and leading object in the cure is, to procure a free passage, by removing or overcoming the spasms and contractions of the bowels, that occasion the obstinate costiveness. Till this can be done, the sick have no relief from their sufferings. If there be no sickness or vomiting, a strong purge is given directly; but that cannot be done if the stomach be irritable and out of order, for without much precaution any purgative, even the gentlest, becomes an emetic. The purgative that was found upon

upon the whole to anfwer beft was, two fcruples of rhubarb, and five grains of *mercurius dulcis* *, made into twelve pills with a little fyrup, of which four were given at a time, and they were repeated every half hour, or every hour, according to the ftate of the ftomach. A fecond quantity, and even a third, were often neceffary, but in that cafe the *mercurius dulcis* was diminifhed, or entirely omitted, left it fhould affect the mouth.

To relieve the pain, fomentations were applied to the abdomen, or recourfe was had to a warm bath. The eafe obtained by thefe means was of fhort duration. A large blifter, applied to that part of the abdomen where the pain was greateft, more effectually procured relief, as foon as it began to rife; and it was further of great ufe in promoting

---

* Calomel, vel Mercurius Muriatus mitis, Pharm. Lond. 1788.

the operation of the purgative, for in general it was obferved, that foon after the pain became eafier free evacuations followed.

Purgative clyfters were thrown up from time to time, in order to promote the operation of the purgative. Of the various compofitions ufed for this purpofe, none appeared better than a folution of common falt in water, confifting of half an ounce, or even a whole ounce to a pint of water. The addition of other articles, often confidered as more ftimulating, appeared to do but little good.

If there were much vomiting or retching, warm water, or an infufion of chamomile flowers, was given; and after the ftomach was quieted a little, the purging pills were adminiftered as before, but with the addition of one or two grains of opium, to prevent their being thrown up. If it were neceffary to repeat the pills, the opium was omitted in a second or third quantity.

In general, by the means already mentioned, stools were procured, and the disease was overcome; yet this was not always the case, for the pain and costiveness would sometimes remain, after every thing recommended above had been carefully put in practice. Under such circumstances recourse was had to other purgatives, as jalap, the *extractum catharticum* *, the purging salts, and the *oleum ricini*. It may seem that some of these, as the jalap, and *extractum catharticum* should have had a trial before the rhubarb and *calomel*, as they are known to be more powerful purgatives. But those substances appear to have their virtues much impaired by keeping, in a warm climate; for they were found not to

* Extract. Colocynthidis comp. Pharm. Lond. 1788.

possess the same strength as in Europe. The rhubarb also is less powerful, but with the addition of the calomel it formed a purge, which more commonly than any other had the desired effect. When this failed, of the purgatives mentioned above, the purging salts were perhaps the best, if the state of the stomach admitted of their use. An ounce and an half of bitter purging salt * were dissolved in three gills of water, to which were added a drachm and a half of the *spiritus lavendulæ compositus*, and three drops of the oil of peppermint, and of this three or four table spoonfuls were given every half hour. The castor oil was a good medicine, when the stomach would retain it; a table spoonful was given for a dose, in a little broth, and it was repeated every hour. It may be observed in general, that whatever purgative was em-

* Magnesia Vitriolata, Pharm. Lond. 1788.

ployed, regard was not had to the common dofe, which would not have been ftrong enough; but it was repeated from time to time, either till it difagreed with the ftomach, or till it operated.

If the pulfe became quick from the violence of the pain and the feverity of the difeafe, provided it were the firft attack, and the patient were full and plethoric, a fmall bleeding, from fix to eight ounces, promoted in feveral inftances the folution of the difeafe.

It became an object of much confequence in the treatment of the colic, to prevent, if poffible, the palfy. That, as far as it could be effected, appeared to depend intirely on the fpeedy cure of the colic; for, the more violent it was, and the longer it continued, the greater reafon was there to fear a palfy would enfue. The remedies, given againft the colic, have fometimes been accufed of producing

producing the paralytic affection; but certainly without foundation. The only effects they could have, either in preventing or producing that stage of the disease, must depend upon their being more or less efficacious in removing the colic.

After the first evacuations by stool were procured, though the strength of the disease was broken, there still remained in many cases a disposition to costiveness, with more or less of pain in the abdomen; for the removal of which, it was proper to give opening medicines from time to time, as the *oleum ricini,* aloetic pills, gum guajacum dissolved in spirits, or any other that agreed with the patient. Those often brought away small balls of hardened *fæces,* several days after the passage of the bowels appeared to have been opened.

Bitters,

Bitters, as an infusion of chamomile flowers, or gentian *, were given to strengthen the stomach.

The second stage of the disease, the palsy, is always a most obstinate complaint, and in many cases the sick never recover completely, either the strength, or motion, of the arms, or wrists. The Bath † waters have long been celebrated for their virtues in this stage of the disease: by bathing in them many have had the use of their limbs restored ‡. There is reason to think, that their good effects depend entirely upon their virtues as a warm bath; and this opinion has been confirmed, by such trials as I have made

---

* Infusum gentianæ comp. Pharm. Lond. 1788.

† There is in the parish of St. Thomas's in the East, in the island of Jamaica, a warm mineral water of nearly the same temperature as the waters of Bath in Somersetshire. The heat of it is about 123° of Fahrenheit, and it is extremely beneficial in the palsy.

‡ Vid. Charlton on Bath waters.

of the warm bath, in the cure of the palsy. It was nearly as effectual as the Bath waters; but the difficulty of preserving a proper and uniform degree of heat, in an artificial warm bath, for any length of time, must always give a decided preference to natural warm springs. It may frequently happen however that those cannot be come at, in which case warm bathing forms an excellent substitute. The temperature of the sea, near the shore in the West Indies, is not less than 84° about the middle of the day, and bathing in it would probably be as efficacious in the cure of palsy as the Bath waters. But in this particular my experience is very limited, for the paralytic men were all sent home with the invalids, as there was hardly a chance of their ever being again fit for soldiers.

There was frequently much pain in the paralytic limbs, and at times puffy swellings

lings in particular parts, which appeared and difappeared fuddenly. Both thofe fymptoms were relieved by the *linimentum volatile* *; and when the pains were violent, eafe was procured by opiates.

In fome few cafes the pain in the bowels fhifted fuddenly to the head, the mifery of the patient became extreme, and in one inftance a temporary madnefs enfued. In this ftate nothing procures equal relief with blifters, applied to the back, behind the ears, and to the temples, fucceffively, as the violence or duration of the pain may require. Opiates alfo procure a flight mitigation of the fufferings of the fick.

I fhall conclude thefe obfervations, with fome remarks on the remedies ufually recommended in this difeafe. The French †, among whom the difeafe is

---

* Linimentum Ammoniæ, Pharm. Lond. 1788.
† Vid. Med. Tranf. vol. ii. p. 459.

frequent, give emetic tartar; but in all the examples of the disease that have fallen under my observation, the vomiting was a troublesome symptom, and a great impediment to the cure; and therefore whatever was likely to excite it, was carefully avoided. The practice would appear to be bad, but as I have no experience of it, I dare not decide upon its merits.

Physicians have been much divided with respect to the use of opiates in this disease; some of great note advise, to trust chiefly to them in the cure of the colic, asserting that they allay the pain, remove the spasms of the bowels, and contribute greatly to a speedy solution of the disease, by rendering the operation of purgatives more easy and certain; while others, of no less name, entirely forbid the use of opiates, till a free passage has been procured. I must own that my experience, as well in this country

country as in Jamaica, coincides with the latter opinion. The relief procured by opiates was inconsiderable, till the body was opened, and some of the worst cases that I saw had been treated with opiates in the beginning. A desire to allay the excruciating pain is the cause that they are frequently given; but the only circumstances under which I have found them of advantage were, when the stomach was very irritable, and they were united to a purgative, to prevent it from being thrown up.

It is not probably of much consequence what purgative is given, provided it operate effectually. In this country the *extractum catharticum* * with the *mercurius dulcis,* and if necessary a small proportion of opium, are very effectual; and I prefer a composition of this kind to the rhubarb and *mercurius dulcis.* Half

* Extractum Colocynthidis compositum, Pharm. Lond. 1788.

a drachm

a drachm of the extract, with five grains of calomel, and a grain and a half of opium, are made into eight pills, of which two are given every hour, or every two hours, according to the state of the stomach, till they operate. A second quantity is often consumed, and sometimes a third, in both of which the opium is generally omitted, before an evacuation is procured. The calomel could not be given so freely in the West Indies, for five grains of it were oftener than once productive of much inconvenience, by exciting salivation, with considerable swelling, pain, and inflammation about the mouth and throat. The constitution in that climate is peculiarly sensible to the effects of mercury, contrary to what might have been expected, were the opinions usually entertained on this subject true; for, if a determination of the humours to the skin could prevent mercury from affecting the mouth, it ought to to be a difficult thing to excite a salivation in Jamaica, where the perspiration is at all times profuse.

Clysters of various kinds were made use of at different times. Warm water with some oil relieved the strangury. Common salt was more stimulating than either the Glauber's, or bitter purging salt. Some trials were made of throwing up the smoke of tobacco, but the dreadful sickness it occasioned, so much aggravated the sufferings of the patient, that it was laid aside, perhaps before we had found out the best manner of managing it.

SECT. III. *Of the Causes of the Dry-Belly-Ach.*

IT will not be deemed necessary, to enter into any detail on this part of the subject,

subject, after what I have advanced in another place *.

That lead taken into the body, in all its various forms, produces colic and palsy, is a fact as well established as any in physic. Nor is it material whether the lead be in vapour, as among smelters; in a metallic state, as among glaziers and plumbers; in a calx, as among painters, and the manufacturers of white lead; or in a saline state, as in wine and cyder: under every form it is equally productive of the disease in question. The quantity of lead requisite to produce the disease admits of considerable variation, for there are clear proofs of its arising from a few grains of Saccharum Saturni †, and also well authenticated cases, in which that salt has been given liberally, and without any immediate ill effect. But what is to be inferred from

---

* Med. Transf. vol. iii. p. 227.
† Med. Transf. vol. i. p. 304.

this more, than that there are some constitutions affected in a shorter time, and by a smaller quantity of this poison, than others * ? An observation applicable not only to every poison, but every active medicine, with which we are acquainted.

That the dry-belly-ach is the effect of lead, some how introduced into the body, cannot reasonably be doubted; and the new rum, distilled in improper vessels, appears to be the vehicle in which it finds admission. I have not yet met with any facts or observations, to induce me to change the opinion I advanced on this subject. It were to be wished however that the matter were prosecuted further, by examining the rum as it comes from the still, and also by ascertaining the contents of the sediment that is found in the vessels, in which

* Med. Transf. vol. i. p. 257. vol. ii. p. 419.

new rum has been kept some time. Such inquiries cannot so well be made in this country as in the West Indies.

I cannot deny myself the pleasure of inserting in this place, a letter from Dr. Franklin to his friend Mr. Vaughan, in which the opinion I have advanced, respecting the cause of the colic in the West Indies, is illustrated and confirmed in some degree, by what happened in New England. Though several of the facts mentioned in the letter are already before the public, I have not chosen either to abridge it, or give it in other words than those, in which the doctor so clearly expresses himself.

Philadelphia, July 31, 1786.

" Dear Friend,
" I recollect that when I had the great
" pleasure of seeing you at Southamp-
† " ton,

" ton, now a twelvemonth since, we
" had some conversation on the bad ef-
" fects of lead taken inwardly; and
" that at your request I promised to send
" you in writing a particular account of
" several facts I then mentioned to you,
" of which you thought some good use
" might be made. I now sit down to
" fulfil that promise.

" The first thing I remember of this
" kind, was a general discourse in Boston
" when I was a boy, of a complaint from
" North Carolina against New England
" rum, that it poisoned their people,
" giving them the dry-belly-ach, with
" a loss of the use of their limbs. The
" distilleries being examined on the oc-
" casion, it was found that several of
" them used leaden still-heads and worms,
" and the physicians were of opinion that
" the mischief was occasioned by that
" use of lead. The legislature of the
" Massachusetts

"Maſſachuſſetts thereupon paſſed an
"act, prohibiting, under ſevere penalties,
"the uſe of ſuch ſtill-heads and worms
"thereafter.

"In 1724, being in London, I went
"to work in the printing-houſe of
"Mr. Palmer, Bartholomew-Cloſe, as a
"compoſitor. I there found a practice,
"I had never ſeen before, of drying a
"caſe of types, (which are wet in diſtri-
"bution) by placing it ſloping before
"the fire. I found this had the addi-
"tional advantage, when the types were
"not only dried but heated, of being
"comfortable to the hands working
"over them in cold weather. I there-
"fore ſometimes heated my caſe when
"the types did not want drying. But
"an old workman obſerving it, adviſed
"me not to do ſo, telling me I might
"loſe the uſe of my hands by it, as two
"of our companions had nearly done,
"one

" one of whom that used to earn his
" guinea a week could not then make
" more than ten shilling, and the other,
" who had the dangles, but seven and
" sixpence. This, with a kind of ob-
" scure pain that I had sometimes felt as
" it were in the bones of my hand when
" working over the types made very hot,
" induced me to omit the practice. But
" talking afterwards with Mr. James,
" a letter-founder in the same Close, and
" asking him if his people, who work-
" ed over the little furnaces of melted
" metal, were not subject to that dis-
" order; he made light of any danger
" from the effluvia, but ascribed it to
" particles of the metal swallowed with
" their food by slovenly workmen, who
" went to their meals after handling the
" metal, without well washing their
" fingers, so that some of the metalline
" particles were taken off by their bread,
" and eaten with it. This appeared to
" have

"have some reason in it. But the pain
"I had experienced made me still afraid
"of those effluvia.

"Being in Derbyshire at some of the
"furnaces for smelting of lead ore, I
"was told that the smoke of those fur-
"naces was pernicious to the neigh-
"bouring grass and other vegetables;
"but I do not recollect to have heard
"any thing of the effect of such vegeta-
"bles eaten by animals. It may be well
"to make the enquiry.

"In America I have often observed
"that on the roofs of our shingled houses,
"where moss is apt to grow in northern
"exposures, if there be any thing on the
"roof painted with white lead, such
"as balusters, or frames of dormant
"windows, &c. there is constantly a
"streak on the shingles from such paint
"down to the eaves, on which no moss
"will grow, but the wood remains con-
"stantly clean and free from it. We sel-
"dom

" dom drink rain-water that falls on our
" houses; and if we did, perhaps the
" small quantity of lead descending from
" such paint, might not be sufficient to
" produce any sensible ill effect on our
" bodies. But I have been told of a
" case in Europe, I forget the place,
" where a whole family was afflicted
" with what we call the dry-belly-ach,
" or *colica pictorum*, by drinking rain-
" water. It was at a country seat, which
" being situated too high to have the
" advantage of a well, was supplied with
" water from a tank which received the
" water from the leaded roofs. This
" had been drank several years without
" mischief; but some young trees plant-
" ed near the house, growing up above
" the roof, and shedding their leaves up-
" on it, it was supposed that an acid in
" those leaves had corroded the lead they
" covered, and furnished the water of
" that

"that year with its baneful particles and qualities.

"When I was in Paris with Sir John Pringle in 1767, he visited *La Charité*, an hospital particularly famous for the cure of that malady, and brought from thence a pamphlet, containing a list of the names of persons, specifying their professions or trades, who had been cured there. I had the curiosity to examine that list, and found that all the patients were of trades that some way or other use or work in lead; such as plumbers, glaziers, painters, &c. excepting only two kinds, stone-cutters and soldiers. In them, I could not reconcile to my notion that lead was the cause of that disorder. But on my mentioning this difficulty to a physician of that hospital, he informed me that the stone-cutters are continually using melted lead to fix the ends of iron balustrades in "stone;

" ftone; and that the foldiers had been
" employed by painters as labourers in
" grinding of colours.

" This, my dear friend, is all I can at
" prefent recollect on the fubject. You
" will fee by it, that the opinion of this
" mifchievous effect from lead, is at leaft
" above fixty years old; and you will
" obferve with concern how long a ufe-
" ful truth may be known, and exift, be-
" fore it is generally received and prac-
" tifed on.

  " I am, ever,

   " Yours moft affectionately,

    " B. FRANKLIN."

The law above alluded to forbids the ufe of leaden heads or worms, under proper penalties; it further prohibits the artificers who make fuch from ufing using any lead in their composition; and it appoints assay-masters, with power to examine and report upon all heads and worms, employed in the distillation of rum, or spirits *.

* The act was passed in 1723 (10 G. I. c. 2.)

CHAP.

CHAP. VI.

Of SORES *and* ULCERS.

SORES and ulcers in the lower extremities were frequent at all seasons of the year, and in all the different quarters where the soldiers were stationed. They, together with fevers and fluxes, amounted to 19-20ths of the sick received into the hospitals, all other complaints not being more than 1-20th, if particular times be excepted, when the colic or small-pox were prevalent. The proportion of sores in the hospitals, though always considerable, admitted of great variation. At Spanish Town and Kingston they were often 1-3d, at Fort-Augusta

gusta 1-half, and at Stoney Hill 2-3ds of the whole number in hospital. They arise from the most trifling causes; a scratch, an hurt, or bruise in the lower extremities, are sufficient to produce a sore, which it is always difficult to heal, and sometimes impossible. Old sores often break out anew, and prove equally obstinate.

A common cause of sores is an insect called a *chiger* *. It is of the flea kind, and extremely small. It lays its eggs in the skin in an uncommon manner, for it is said to bury itself in the flesh, and become a *nidus* for its own *ova*. The part, where it has thus deposited itself, after a little time swells, becomes red, and itches much. At this period, it is the common practice, to pick out of the skin with a fine needle the bag formed by the body of the parent insect, in which are contained the rudiments of the young. If this be neglected, the inflammation in-

* Pulex penetrans, Linnæi Syst. Nat.

creases,

creafes, fuppuration takes place, and an ulcer is formed. The infect harbours moft commonly in duft upon the floor or ground, and generally depofits its *ova* in the toes and feet; and many of the men loft one or more of their toes, by ulcers arifing from this caufe.

Sores, in whatever way produced, fpread quickly, and form a large ulcrated furface. They give little or no pain, which appears to be owing in a great degree to the warmth of the air, for cuts and wounds are found to give much lefs pain in a warm, than in a cold climate. The appearances of the ulcers are conftantly varying; at times they acquire the look of an healthy fore, fend forth ftrong and luxuriant granulations, and begin to fkin over; but one night will often put an end to this flattering profpect. The granulations turn flaccid, or even mortify in part, the portion fkinned over ulcerates afrefh, and the fore becomes larger than ever. After a time it will again put on an healing appearance, and repeatedly run through the same stages. The bones at last become carious, and if the limb be not either amputated, or the patient sent off the island, he becomes hectic, and after lingering a considerable time, dies.

The extreme difficulty, indeed almost impossibility, of healing an ulcer in the lower extremities, after it had become of a certain size, necessarily produced an accumulation of such cases in the hospitals. Various means of cure were attempted, the principal of which it will be sufficient to mention shortly, as none of them were attended with considerable success.

It was supposed, as the soldiers arrived in the island after being a long time at sea, and as they had salt provisions after landing, that they might have more or less of scurvy in their habit, which would

would render the ulcers difficult of cure. On this suppofition they were put upon a vegetable diet, which for a time had good effects upon some, but in the end failed.

The powers of the conftitution having evidently fuffered, it was imagined they might be reftored by the use of bark, with a full and nourifhing diet. This plan was accordingly tried, and produced at firft favourable changes, but was not finally more fuccefsful than the former.

Alterative medicines, as fmall dofes of calomel, were given, but they did no good. The changes, which the ulcers of themfelves underwent, occafioned for a while, fome degree of deception as to the good effects of the treatment made use of; for the favourable appearances of the ulcers, coinciding as to time with the medicines directed, raifed expectations at firft, which, in the end, were difappointed.

But

But it muſt be allowed, that in many caſes the means employed produced a temporary amendment, and promoted to a certain degree the efforts of nature to effect a cure; yet the powers of the conſtitution were ſo feeble, that with all the aſſiſtance that could be given, they could not bring it to a completion. They advanced a certain way, but ſoon fell back again.

External applications of various kinds were tried, and what has been ſaid of the internal remedies will equally apply to them; they often produced a favourable change at firſt, but it was not permanent. Among the different dreſſings that were made trial of were ointments, ſometimes ſtimulating, ſometimes emollient, fermenting poultices, the common bread and milk poultice, and dry lint. An application common among the inhabitants deſerves to be taken notice of, as it ſometimes had better effects than any

any of those just mentioned, I mean roasted limes.

An horizontal position with quiet did good as in other countries, and if neglected the progress of ulcers became extremely rapid.

The general result of all my experience was, that ulcers of some standing, and of a considerable size, in the lower extremities, could not be healed in that country by any means that we were acquainted with. Instead therefore of wasting time in fruitless trials, every opportunity was taken of sending home the men with ulcers, along with the other invalids. The change of air and climate produced great effects; many of the ulcers healed on the passage, and all of them soon got well after their arrival in England, unless where the bones were carious; and of these last many recovered, after losing large portions of the *tibia* by exfoliations, or were finally restored to health,

by

by an amputation of the difeafed limb. This operation was indeed fometimes performed in Jamaica, but never except under the moft urgent circumftances, for it feldom fucceeded, owing to the locked jaw, which generally came on in a few days, and proved fatal. I cannot help therefore concluding, that humanity as well as the good of the fervice require, that all bad ulcers fhould be fent home without lofs of time from the Weft Indies, unlefs fome more effectual means of cure fhould be difcovered, than thofe with which we are hitherto acquainted.

Although ulcers can feldom be cured in the Weft Indies, they may often be prevented. The chigers get to the toes and feet by the men going without fhoes or ftockings; who, from the fame caufe are alfo more expofed to fcratches and bruifes in thofe parts, which quickly become ulcers, if not treated directly with great attention. If care were taken,

that

that they should never go without shoes and stockings, or trowsers in the room of stockings, it would prevent many ulcers, particularly at Stoney Hill, where the chigers are very numerous, though in other respects it be the most healthy quarter in the island. At Fort-Augusta, Port-Royal, and other quarters near the sea, the men in fishing or wading in the water for their amusement, often cut their feet upon the stones and rocks, and so give rise to ulcers, which it would not be difficult to prevent.

CHAP. VII.

Of some other Diseases to which Soldiers are subject.

OF the following diseases, which all together form a very inconsiderable proportion of the sick list, there are few peculiarities, either in their history or treatment, depending upon the climate; yet such as there are, I thought it might not be without use to take notice of shortly.

Sect. I. *Of the Venereal Disease.*

OF the few things peculiar to this disease, in the West Indies, it is perhaps the most singular, that it should, at the present

present day, be much less frequent in a country supposed originally to have produced it, than in any part of Europe. This will not be considered as a proof, that the venereal disease had its origin in the West Indies. In 331 patients admitted into the hospital of the 92d regiment, there were only two with venereal complaints; and in the other hospitals, the disease was not more frequent. Though less common than in Europe, it is not milder; on the contrary the proportion of cases, in which the disease is violent and the symptoms run high, is greater. This is probably to be imputed to the bad habit of body, which not only makes it difficult to heal sores in the extremities, but also renders the progress of inflammation in many cases unfavourable, and tedious. In gonorrhœa, the inflammation of the urethra often extends to the bladder, producing strangury, and the usually concomitant symptoms.

Chancres

Chancres often produce *phimosis* and *paraphimosis*, and consequent mortification. Such unfavourable symptoms are found to happen in patients, who are of a bad habit of body, in all countries. In one case the venereal blotches ulcerated, and three or four large sores were formed upon the arms and shoulders, which could not be healed by any means that were tried; they remained after there was reason to believe, that all traces of the infection were eradicated. The patient was sent home to England, and soon after he sailed, the sores began to heal, and were all well before he arrived at an end of the voyage.

The great sensibility of the constitution to the effects of mercury, in the West Indies, often proves a considerable obstacle to the cure of this disease. A salivation is frequently excited, before a sufficient quantity of the medicine can be thrown in. Bark, in the quantity of three or four drachms

drachms a day, and the free ufe of opiates, together with an aftringent gargle, made of a decoction of oak bark, to which fome alum may be added, prevent the mouth from being either fo quickly, or fo violently affected. Of the feveral preparations of mercury, the *mercurius calcinatus* * was found to be the beft for internal ufe.

It is worth remarking, that mercury had no effect upon the conftitution to render it lefs fufceptible of fevers; for perfons under a courfe of that medicine were feized with the remittent fever; which however did not appear to be aggravated by the prefence of the mercury in the body.

* Hydrargyrus calcinatus, Pharm. Lond. 1788.

SECT.

Sect. II. *Of some Complaints arising from Insects.*

BESIDES the chiger, there are other insects that produce very troublesome complaints, and none perhaps occasion greater distress than musquitoes*. They breed in water, and of course low marshy grounds, and their neighbourhood, are particularly infested by them. They are most troublesome in the morning and evening, during the calm that takes place between the land and sea breezes; they dislike the wind. Their bite produces violent itching, inflammation, and sometimes sores in consequence of scratching, from which it is difficult to refrain. When the proboscis of a musquito is examined with a microscope, it is found to consist of a sheath contain-

* Culex pipiens, Linnæi Syst. Nat.

ing

ing small pointed bristles, with which it penetrates the skin while it sucks, and when the insect is brushed off suddenly, they are probably in part broken, and remain sticking in the skin, and thereby contribute greatly to produce the tormenting itching, that is the consequence of the bite of those insects, and which is always aggravated by scratching.

Lime juice, or rum, are the applications commonly made use of, and they both allay the itching. A mixture of them, in equal parts, appeared to be more efficacious than either separately. It has been proposed by a writer *, who has examined the history of this insect with the greatest accuracy, to wash the face and hands, or such parts as are exposed to the bites of musquitoes, with the juice or decoction of certain herbs, which might possibly prevent them en-

* Reaumur, Hist. des Insects, vol. iv. p. 624.

tirely from making their attacks upon the skin. It is probable experiments might in this way discover the complete means of prevention, and among other applications deserving of trial, the writer above referred to, recommends an infusion of pepper, wormwood, or rue; verjuice, pomatums, &c.

There is a large fly that produces often a dreadful disease, by depositing its ova in the mouth or nose. It happens frequently to negroes, and we had several examples of it among the common soldiers. While they are sleeping in the open air, the fly deposits its ova most commonly in the nose, but sometimes in the mouth. The pain, swelling, and inflammation about the face, after the maggots are formed and ready to break forth, are very great; and the poor sufferers are almost distracted. The number of living maggots that come away is often considerable, and they are of a

large

large size, being nearly half an inch long.

The usual remedy in such cases is, inhaling the steam of a strong decoction of the leaves of tobacco, through the mouth or nose, according to the seat of the disease. It procures great relief. The tobacco is used on the supposition that it kills the maggots, but whether the good effects of it depend upon any power of that kind, or simply on the vapour and steam, I did not see a sufficient number of cases to determine. If the virtues of the tobacco have a considerable share in the cure, it is probable that a weaker decoction or infusion of the leaves, thrown up the nose by a syringe, or used to wash the mouth with from time to time, would prove more effectual in destroying the maggots than the vapour or steam.

WHILE speaking of the diseases produced by insects, it will not be out of place

place to mention some singularities respecting the itch, a disease which arises from a particular species of insect*. It has been doubted whether this disorder really depends upon an insect, but I have frequently seen them picked out of the skin, and examined them with a microscope. They were first observed by *Bonomo* †, and the figure given by him conveys a tolerable idea of the insect.

In this country the itch commonly appears between the fingers, about the wrists, and in such parts of the body, as by a duplicature of the skin, are in some degree defended from the action of the air, and are of course warmer than the other parts. But this is not the case in the West Indies; the disease spreads almost uniformly over the skin, which is probably to be imputed to the heat of the climate. In a temperature of the air

* Acarus siro, Linnæi Syst. Nat.
† Phil. Transf. vol. xxiii. p. 1296. an. 1703.

between 80° and 90°, the infect is not impelled to feek for fhelter in the folds of the fkin.

The itch is a diforder productive in general of effects, which, though troublefome and difagreeable, can feldom be called dangerous; yet in certain fituations I have feen it occafion alarming fymptoms, which have fo far difguifed the difeafe, that it could not for a time be known to be the itch. The fmall pointed watery veficle, or puftule, which characterifes the itch, has been changed into an eating fore, that in part deftroyed the fubftance of the fkin. Such effects, it was not at firft imagined, could arife from the itch; but when it was obferved to infect others, and produce in them the common appearances of the difeafe, it occafioned a fufpicion of the nature of the complaint, which was confirmed by the readinefs with which all the fymptoms yielded to the external application of fulphur. I have never seen the effects of the itch just mentioned, except in children, and those under the following circumstances; either in the confined apartments of a workhouse, where children are always unhealthy; or where, by mistake, the disease has been allowed to remain a long time, in consequence of which ulcers have been formed, the sleep broken, and the general health greatly impaired. Under all circumstances, however, the cure is equally easy and certain, for the disease yields as readily to the sulphur ointment, when attended with the unusual symptoms, as in its more common form.

Sect. III. *Of Inflammatory Disorders.*

INFLAMMATORY diseases are very rare in Jamaica, though not always slight when

when they do occur. Catarrhs, coughs, inflammations of the breaſt, and of the lungs, are uncommon; yet in the months of March and April, when there is the greateſt difference between the temperature of the air in the day and in the night, they are ſometimes to be met with; and oftener at Spaniſh Town than Kingſton. Several of the ſoldiers were ſeized with inflammations of the breaſt, in conſequence of a ſtorm of wind and rain, which happened in the night-time at Spaniſh Town, and by deſtroying part of the roof of the barracks, expoſed the men to the cold and wet. One of them died, and the others recovered ſlowly; for, though the diſeaſe was ſoon overcome by bleeding and the uſual remedies, yet it was a conſiderable time before they regained their ſtrength, which was probably to be imputed to the neceſſary loſs of blood.

Inflammations of the eyes are frequent, obſtinate,

obstinate, and full of danger, for they often terminate in opacities of the *cornea*. The glare and heat of the sun, strongly reflected by the ground, devoid at certain seasons of verdure; and the dust rendered light and dry by heat, and put in motion by the trade wind, which often blows with violence during part of the day; are to be considered as the causes of the frequent inflammations of the eyes.

The bad habit of body, that prevails almost universally among Europeans, renders such inflammations obstinate, and in the end productive of opacities, and loss of sight. Having before mentioned a bad habit of body, and assigned it as a cause why ulcers in the lower extremities are so easily produced, and healed with so much difficulty; and having again considered it as the cause, which renders inflammations of the eyes obstinate, and productive of the worst consequences; it may

may be afked wherein this bad habit of body confifts, in order that too much may not be afcribed to a caufe, of which we have only a vague or ill-defined idea? To this I would anfwer, that the bad habit of body fhews itfelf chiefly in a weaknefs of the powers of nature, in healing even trifling fores from external injuries, and alfo in the readinefs with which inflammation of all kinds takes an unfavourable courfe. The powers of life, upon which the repair and fupport of the fimple folids of the body depend, appear to be weakened, though there be no evident diminution either of mufcular ftrength, or animal fpirits. It may be a queftion, whether this weaknefs depend upon the heat of the climate, which at firft produces a great fenfe of laffitude from the fmalleft exertions, and may ftill operate unfavourably upon the body, after time and habit have got over the firft difagreeable feelings: or, whether it it arise from the cause of fever, which prevails more or less at all times of the year, and may therefore operate insensibly on the constitution, without producing the disease; like to what sometimes happens in the jail fever [*]. Facts and observations might be produced, some in favour of, and others adverse to, each of the opinions above stated. It is not improbable, that there may be some foundation for both; but I forbear to enter farther on a subject, on which I am not provided with materials, from whence any certain conclusions can be drawn.

Inflammations of the eyes, having often fatal terminations, ought not for a moment to be neglected, even though trifling at first; and the means, usually employed against such complaints, should be put in practice with the utmost diligence. It would be superfluous to enter into a detail upon this head, for I have not learned any thing peculiar to

[*] Med. Tranf. vol. iii. p. 357.

the treatment of the difeafe in that country.

The common fore throat occurs now and then, and is almoft always a flight difeafe.

It may deferve to be taken notice of, that the meafles is commonly a mild difeafe in Jamaica. It was frequent among the Duke of Cumberland's regiment in 1782-3, which confifted of Americans, of whom many had never had that difeafe. Few of them were fo ill as to be taken into the hofpital, and in thofe the fever was very flight; and none of them were troubled either with complaints of their breaft, or bowels, the ufual concomitants or confequences of the meafles. The difeafe appeared to be greatly mitigated by the warmth of the climate, which leffened the difpofition to inflammation, particularly in the breaft. Something analogous to this is to be obferved in England; the meafles are milder in the

the warmer months, and are much less apt to affect the breast dangerously at such times, than in the winter or spring. From some few cases however that fell under my observation among the inhabitants, the measles may become a formidable disease, in consequence of a subsequent dysentery. Under those circumstances, the practice so strongly recommended by Sydenham, that is bleeding, will rarely, if ever, be admissible in patients, whose constitutions are exhausted both by the climate and the disease. The alternate use of opening medicines and opiates, as recommended in treating of the dysentery, succeeded well; and there was room for employing astringents sooner than in common cases of dysentery.

SECT. IV. *Of Confumptions, Mania, and Prickly Heat.*

PULMONARY confumptions rarely originate in the ifland, but thofe who come from England with that complaint already begun, are not benefited by the warmth of the climate; on the contrary, the difeafe is precipitated, and proves fooner fatal than it would have done in a more temperate air. Of this we had repeated examples among the foldiers, feveral of whom arrived in the ifland with beginning confumptions, and were all quickly carried off by that difeafe.

It deferves to be mentioned, that feveral examples of *mania* occurred among the troops. In fuch cafes as fell immediately under my obfervation, the difeafe was evidently owing to an intemperate ufe of fpirituous liquors; and fome,
while

while they could be prevailed upon to abstain from spirits, were in a great measure free from the disease; but others, after being once attacked, continued for years to labour under that deplorable distemper.

Before I dismiss this subject, I may be permitted to take notice of a disease, if so trifling an affection deserve that name, that is very common, I mean the *prickly heat*. Some are troubled with it all the year round; others only during the warmer months. Such as have fair and delicate complexions are more subject to it than others, insomuch that they are not free from it at times either night or day. Some are incommoded by it only when exposed to the heat of the sun, or on making bodily exertions.

The prickly heat consists of a small red rash, chiefly upon such parts of the skin as are covered. It scarcely appears to the eye to be raised above the skin, though

though it gives it a flight roughnefs to the feel. It is attended with a difagreeable fenfation of heat and pricking in the fkin, as is well expreffed by its name. It is fuppofed by fome to be a falutary effort of the conftitution, and the difappearance of it is therefore dreaded as portending mifchief. I cannot fay that I ever met with any facts to confirm this opinion. In the beginning of fevers, it is common for it to difappear, if they are preceded by a chilly or cold fit, and to return again with the hot fit, but without appearing in either cafe to aggravate, or alleviate the difeafe.

The prickly heat probably depends upon a two-fold caufe; the irritating action of the heat upon the fkin, and the concentrated ftate of the falts in the perfpirable matter. The rays of the fun in warm climates are capable even of raifing blifters on the fkin; and the perfpiration always being profufe, the thinner parts soon fly off, and the remainder becomes more loaded with the animal salts, and is of course more irritating.

It requires no medicine, and the troublesome effects arising from it, are best remedied, or prevented, by quiet and rest.

CHAP. VIII.

Remarks on some of the Diseases of NEGROES.

THE diseases of negroes fell seldom under my observation; what I have to say of them therefore will be very short, and chiefly with a view of calling the attention of others to the subject: for we are hitherto much in the dark respecting several disorders, that are in a great measure confined to the negroes, in that part of the world. A better history of them would enlarge our knowledge of pathology, and teach us, I doubt not, many new and interesting facts in the animal œconomy. It is much to be regretted, that a work of this kind is not attempted by some of the profession in

Jamaica or our other West India islands, in which there are many men of observation every way equal to such an undertaking.

The *yaws* is perhaps one of the most remarkable diseases, that prevail among negroes. It is infectious, and, like the small-pox, never attacks a person a second time. It is communicated by contact, most commonly in the same way that the venereal disease is; for it is seldom caught without some close connection, or intimate communication. It is distinguished by numerous superficial sores of no great size, in each of which are small spherical prominences, in appearance like a raspberry. There is general soreness, and lassitude at their first eruption, but no fever. The discharge from the sores is more of a slimy mucus than matter. The length of the disease is various, extending from four or five, to fifteen or twenty months. If a negro, that has

has contracted the diforder, be put in circumftances favourable to general health; if he be not obliged to work, if he be allowed a good diet, and if he be kept clean by frequent wafhings, it will run its courfe, and after a time entirely difappear. We are not acquainted with any means of eradicating the poifon, for though mercurials will put an entire ftop to the difeafe, nay remove every morbid appearance, yet it is only for a time: the difeafe is fufpended, not fubdued, and it foon recurs again. It is the opinion of fome, that there is much danger from thus interrupting the courfe of the difeafe by mercury, and that it becomes afterwards more obftinate and productive of new diforders, as violent pains, known under the name of the *bone-ach*. Some admit the ufe of mercury, provided it be not early in the difeafe, and fay that the diforder does not then return. The period of the difeafe, when it can be given with benefit, is not ascertained with any degree of precision.

Respecting this disease there are many *desiderata*; we are unacquainted with the local effects of the poison when it is first applied, and also with the interval of time, between the application and the first appearance of the disease upon the skin. Both those points would be ascertained by inoculation, a practice which has been proposed, and appears to be well deserving of a trial, in this disorder. It would be of great consequence to ascertain, the earliest period at which mercury might be given with advantage. The bone-ach, and other disorders, the effects either real or supposed of the yaws, are undescribed. These are some of the most obvious heads of inquiry on this subject.

The yaws is a disorder not peculiar to negroes, for several of the soldiers were affected with it.

Cacabay

Cacabay is a negro name for a difease not known among Europeans or their defcendants, as far as I could learn. It begins in whitifh fpots upon the fkin, near the ends of the extremities. Thofe fpots turn to ulcers commonly upon the fingers and toes; there is much fwelling with pain, and the joint affected drops off, without any mortification. The fore afterwards heals up, and remains well even for months; but returns again, affects the next joint, which after a time drops off; and the difease, attacking one joint after another, in the end reduces the miferable fufferer to a mere trunk. It continues often feveral years before it prove fatal.

No remedy has been found either to cure it, or much retard its progrefs. Mercurials have been tried, but with little or no advantage. It were greatly to be wifhed, that the fymptoms of a difease fo formidable and fo fingular, were detailed at full length.

The last disease I shall mention is no less singular than either of the preceding, and much more frequent and destructive. It appears to be more a disorder of the mind than of the body, and shews itself by a very uncommon depravity of the appetite in *eating dirt*. Dirt-eaters, as they are called, can seldom or ever be corrected of this unnatural practice, for their attachment to it is greater, than even that of dram-drinkers to their pernicious liquor. They have a predilection for particular kinds of earth at first, but in the end will eat plaster from the walls, or dust collected from the floor, when they can come at no other. They are fondest of a kind of white clay, like tobacco-pipe-clay, with which they fill their mouths, and allow it to dissolve gradually; and express as much satisfaction from it, as the greatest lover of tobacco could do. This practice is common at all ages, even almost as soon as they leave the

the breaft, the young learning it from the old.

Befides the pleafure they have in this practice after it has become habitual, they are fuppofed to give into it at firft from other motives, fuch as difcontent with their prefent fituation, and a defire of death in order to return to their own country, for they are well aware that it will infallibly deftroy them. It is fuppofed, that a difeafed ftate of the ftomach may give rife to the depraved appetite, but of this there is no good evidence; and as was obferved before, it appears to be more a difeafe of the mind than of the body. Whatever the motives may be that induce them to begin the practice, it foon proves fatal if carried to great excefs. There are inftances of their killing themfelves in ten days, but this is uncommon; and they often drag on a miferable exiftence for feveral months, or even one or two years. The fymptoms that it induces are thofe of a dropfy; the appetite fails, the face becomes bloated, the extremities fwell, and effufions of water take place under the fkin, and in all the cavities of the body.

On examining the body after death, there are frequently found in the colon large concretions of the earthy matter, which they have fwallowed, lining the cavity of the gut, and almoft completely obftructing the paffage. The mefenteric glands are always fwelled. The blood is thin, and with few red globules, as is common in dropfies; and there are large *polypi* in the left ventricle of the heart and the aorta. They are very ftrong and firm, and pulled out give the reprefentation of an injection of the aorta, fubclavian, and carotid arteries. In order to afcertain, whether they were formed before or after death, the body has been opened a few minutes after the patient expired, and they have been found already ftrong and firm.

Diseases of Negroes.

firm *. They are no doubt formed, when the motion of the heart becomes feeble and languid, juſt before death.

No means of preventing the horrid practice of *eating dirt*, as it is called, nor any method of remedying the deſtructive effects of it, have hitherto been diſcovered: a negro labouring under the malady is conſidered as loſt. On many eſtates, half the number of the deaths, on a moderate computation, are owing to this cauſe. They are not to be deterred from it by ſtripes, promiſes, or threats; nor have ſtomachic medicines, magneſia and abſorbents, or a good and full diet ever done much good. What could not be effected by any of the means juſt mentioned, has been in part accompliſhed upon ſome eſtates, as I have been informed, by cutting off the heads from the

* The obſervations made upon the dead body were communicated to me by Dr. Thomas Clarke, botaniſt of the iſland of Jamaica.

dead bodies of thofe, who have died of this vicious practice. The negroes have the utmoft horror and dread of their bodies being treated in this manner, and the efficacy of this expedient, which can only operate upon the mind, is a ftrong proof, that the difeafe in its origin is more a mental than a corporeal affection.

CHAP.

CHAP. IX.

Of the best Manner of taking Care of the Sick of Armies in Jamaica, and our other West Indian Islands.

FROM what has been said in the foregoing pages, it must appear that the far greater part of the diseases, to which soldiers are subject in the West Indies, are of such a nature as to require immediate care, and attention. Time lost in procuring admission into a general hospital is irretrievable. It is still worse if the hospital be at a distance, and the sick are to be sent to it; for besides the delay, they are exposed to fatigue, which never fails greatly to aggravate the disease;

ease; and both together diminish in an high degree the chance of recovery. Wherever soldiers are, there also should be the means of taking care of the sick; not only every regiment, but every detachment, should have an hospital. Were the troops to be placed in the healthy quarters already pointed out, as it would greatly reduce the number of sick, so it would be productive of considerable savings both in the quantity of medicines, and in the number of attendants; but till that be done, we must consider them as remaining in their present situation, and requiring suitable provision. The observations I have to make may be arranged under the heads of *attendance, medicines and hospital stores,* and *subsistence.*

There has been occasion to observe, in examining the returns of the sick, that it is no uncommon thing for their number to amount to one third of the whole, and therefore provision should be made for

for that proportion. Fifty sick, supposing fifteen or twenty of them to be convalescents, are as many as one person, whether a regimental surgeon or mate, or an hospital mate, can take care of; and if the proportion of fevers and fluxes among the sick, and the close attention they require be adverted to, it must be allowed that one person should be possessed both of diligence and assiduity, to do justice to that number. At that rate, therefore, there ought to be a surgeon to every 150 men. As there is sometimes more sickness in one regiment than another, it is for the good of the service to have the assistant surgeons upon the staff establishment, and not attached to any particular corps, that they may be moved more readily from place to place, as the number of the sick may require. A surgeon, that would do justice to the men under his care, must be very frequent in his visits to the hospital; for unless he watch assiduously

siduously the remissions of the fever, and be ready to take immediate advantage of them, he will not be able to check the disease speedily, without which both the constitution and life of the patient will be in imminent danger. A man that has three or four fits of the fever, is in greater danger of dying, than one that has only one or two: but laying the risk of death out of the question, a man that has his fever stopped after the first or second fit, will generally be restored to health in a few days, whereas if he have four or five fits, it will often require as many weeks to recover the same degree of strength in the latter case, as days in the former.

It must therefore be obvious, how much the diligence and attention of the surgeon importeth; of which a very striking proof occurred in a regiment, which was strong, and consisted of twelve companies. The regiment was provided with two hospitals and two surgeons, each of whom

whom took charge of the sick of six companies. It was presently found that one hospital was much fuller than the other, which did not appear to proceed from a greater sickness among one division of the companies than the other, for there was no material difference in the number of sick sent from the several companies. In order to bring the sick in the two hospitals to an equality, a company was taken from one division and annexed to the other. The sick of the five companies were, however, still more numerous than that of the seven; and after a short trial, they were divided into four and eight companies, and then the sick in the two hospitals were nearly equal, and varied from forty to sixty in each. It may be supposed, that so great a difference depended upon the method of treatment being entirely different in the two hospitals. That however was not the case; the general plan of treatment was

nearly

nearly the same in both, and not materially different from what has been mentioned in speaking of the cure of the remittent fever [*]. It was owing to the following circumstances: one surgeon visited his hospital four or five times a day, the other only twice a day; the first seldom allowed any remission to pass without taking advantage of it, the latter, often; one was always at hand to palliate the untoward symptoms, as vomitings, or purgings, proceeding either from the medicines or the disease; the other, not. Add to these, that vigilance in the surgeon at the head of an hospital extends itself to the servants, and nurses under him, and thence a greater degree of attention, both in administering nourishment and medicines. The effect of all those causes was, that the men recovered in half the time in one hospital that they

[*] This appeared from the medicines entered in the hospital book, to be taken notice of afterwards.

did

did in the other, and therefore the hofpital for eight companies had no greater number of fick, than that for four.

A book was kept in every hofpital, in which was entered the name of each patient, his age, the time of his admiffion, the difeafe under which he laboured, and the medicines which were daily given to him. This was found equally ufeful and convenient to the furgeons, and to the phyfician or infpector of the hofpitals: and from this book a weekly return was made of the fick admitted, difcharged, and remaining in the hofpital.

I cannot help fuggefting that an hofpital book or regifter, kept in the manner recommended, in each regiment, and on board every fhip of war, would afford the beft proofs of the diligence and abilities of the furgeons; and if annually tranfmitted to thofe, to whofe fuperintendance the care of the health of the navy and army is committed, would have the good effect of making induftry and abilities known at the greateft diftance. A plan of this kind might greatly contribute to improve our knowledge of difeafes, in all the various climates to which the poffeffions of the Britifh empire extend; and, by enabling us to take better care of the health of our feamen and foldiers, prove a national benefit.

The fubfiftence of the fick in *general hofpitals* has always been found extremely expenfive, yet on actual fervice they appear to be indifpenfable. In our Weft-India iflands they are not only unneceffary, but would be pernicious to the troops in garrifon; and the ufe of them was difcontinued in Jamaica, by directions from the infpector general of hofpitals, with the beft effect.

The mode of fubfifting the fick, in regimental hofpitals, muft vary according to local circumftances; in Jamaica it was ordered fo, that while juftice was done to the fick, they were hardly

hardly a greater expence to government than the men who were well. Of the *rations* or provisions issued to the soldiers, bread only was given to the sick. In the room of the salt meat, rum, and other articles, they had five shillings *currency* * a week, which was the value that the commissaries put upon them, and which they paid weekly in lieu of the provisions. To the sum of five shillings per week was added one shilling and eight pence currency, out of the soldiers pay. The subsistence of the sick therefore consisted of the usual allowance of bread, and six shillings and eight pence currency per week. This money was laid out in purchasing fresh meat, vegetables, coffee, sugar, milk, and other articles necessary for the sick. It was amply sufficient for all those purposes, and even for the payment of *orderly* men,

* Five pounds sterling are equal to seven pounds currency.

who acted as nurses; for there were few or no female nurses in any of the hospitals; they ruined their health by drinking, and could not be depended upon so much as the men. An account of the money above specified was kept in a book in the hospital, open to the inspection of the officers of the regiment, and of the physician or inspector of the hospitals. The subsistence of the sick so far cost government no more than that of the men in health; but it was necessary to allow wine as a medicine, and that in considerable quantities; wine therefore and medicines were the only extraordinary hospital expences. For the purchase of wine ample provision was made by the island: and it ought to be mentioned, that the GENERAL ASSEMBLY of Jamaica, both in this and in every thing else appertaining to the accommodation of the troops, shewed at all times a most laudable disposition to make the greatest exertions.

Besides

Besides medicines and wine it was necessary to have among hospital stores, bedding, cooking utensils, and several other articles that are wanted in furnishing an hospital; for soldiers are allowed no bedding in the West Indies, and generally have none except a blanket. Medicines must necessarily be provided by government in that country, for what is called the medicine money of a surgeon, would not purchase one twentieth part of the requisite articles. Bark alone would cost some hundred pounds; it is often sold in the country for three pounds currency *per pound*, and at a moderate computation, one pound annually is necessary for each man. From this article alone a judgment may be formed, how much it is beyond the power either of a surgeon of a ship of war, or of a regiment, to furnish medicines for the men in that country; and unless government interpose, the sick must remain destitute of many

many things, that are often indispensably necessary for their preservation. Ample provision has always been made for the army, and why equal care should not be taken of our brave seamen, it will be difficult to assign any good reason.

It has been an object of principal consideration, in allowing medicines to the army, to prevent the abuse of them. The high value, which they bear in that climate, has been believed in some cases to prove a temptation to those, through whose hands they passed. It is an easy matter to establish proper checks upon the expenditure of medicines, and it was done in this manner. An exact state of the medicines, wine, and other articles in store, was taken; and the storekeeper, purveyor, or other person having charge of them, was directed to issue none without a written order from the physician, inspector of hospitals, or one having authority to give such orders. Those orders, with a receipt upon them

from

from the surgeon of the regiment, or person in whose favour they were granted, were vouchers to the storekeeper. By these means, no abuses could exist without detection; and that they might more easily appear upon the face of the account, a quarterly return of the expenditure of medicines was regularly made. The orders for medicines are necessarily granted by a person, whether physician, or inspector, who superintends the care of the sick in general, and to whom the weekly returns of the sick in hospital are made. He will therefore at all times be a judge of the quantities of medicines necessary for particular regiments or detachments, as the state of their sick must be known to him. If any abuses are suspected to take place, after the medicines come into the hands of the surgeons, or others having charge of the sick, it is an easy matter to ascertain what grounds there are for such suspicions, by examining the hospital book, in which is an account of all medicines ordered for the sick. I should trespass on the patience of my reader, to enter farther in detail upon this subject, where it must be obvious, that the means of preventing, or detecting abuses, are equally simple and effectual.

In consequence of the men being rendered unfit for service, by repeated attacks of fever, flux, dry-belly-ach, and by sores, the number of invalids accumulated daily in the hospitals, and in the regiments. Humanity as well as the interest of government required, that such should be sent home from time to time. While they remained in the island they were a burden upon the army, without any chance of their ever being useful; but upon being sent to a cooler and more healthy climate, many of them recovered; particularly those who were broken down by fevers, or laboured under sores.

F I N I S.

www.ingramcontent.com/pod-product-compliance
Lightning Source LLC
Chambersburg PA
CBHW031852220426
43663CB00006B/592